'*Yoga Games to Teach in Schools* is one of the most
sound books I've read for yoga in primary schools. Michael
suggests a wide range of inclusive, calming, skill-based games
for yoga, designed to be used within curriculum lessons.
The activities will give your pupils a well-deserved boost in
self-esteem and leadership skills, and support a growth mindset
for both physical and mental wellbeing.'

– Ilse Fullarton, PE Consultant, Association for PE East Board
Member and Founder of The Children's Health Project CIC

'All readers, regardless of their background, will find much to
vitalise their thinking in this book. Michael's unique approach to
yoga is accessible to all children, regardless of their needs and
abilities. He has created a fun range of yoga activities to focus and
stimulate young minds.'

– Kate Mason, Assistant Head, Phoenix School, a school for
children with language and communication difficulties whose
needs lie within the autistic spectrum

'This is a wonderful book for yoga teachers and mums and dads
wanting to develop their children in yoga. I particularly liked the
learning outcomes suggesting why the exercises or games would
be useful. I would highly recommend this to my friends with
children, and to other teachers who would like a resource book
with so much for children of all ages to try, and enjoy!'

– Andrea Kwiatkowski, yoga teacher at Santosha Yoga

Yoga Games

to Teach in Schools

by the same author

Seahorse's Magical Sun Sequences
How all children (and sea creatures) can use yoga to feel positive,
confident and completely included
Michael Chissick
Illustrated by Sarah Peacock
ISBN 978 1 84819 283 6
eISBN 978 0 85701 230 2

Ladybird's Remarkable Relaxation
How children (and frogs, dogs, flamingos and dragons)
can use yoga relaxation to help deal with stress, grief,
bullying and lack of confidence
Michael Chissick
Illustrated by Sarah Peacock
ISBN 978 1 84819 146 4
eISBN 978 0 85701 112 1

Frog's Breathtaking Speech
How children (and frogs) can use yoga breathing to deal
with anxiety, anger and tension
Michael Chissick
Illustrated by Sarah Peacock
ISBN 978 1 78775 613 7
eISBN 978 0 85701 074 2

of related interest

Asanas for Autism and Special Needs
Yoga to Help Children with their Emotions, Self-Regulation
and Body Awareness
Shawnee Thornton Hardy
ISBN 978 1 84905 988 6
eISBN 978 1 78450 059 7

Yoga Therapy for Every Special Child
Meeting Needs in a Natural Setting
Nancy Williams
Illustrated by Leslie White
ISBN 978 1 84819 027 6
eISBN 978 0 85701 027 8

Yoga Games

to Teach in Schools

52 Activities to Develop Self-Esteem,
Self-Control and Social Skills

Michael Chissick

Illustrated by Sarah Peacock

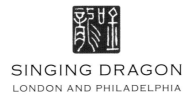

SINGING DRAGON
LONDON AND PHILADELPHIA

First edition published as *Sitting on a Chicken* in Great Britain in 2017
by Singing Dragon, an imprint of Jessica Kingsley Publishers

This edition published in Great Britain in 2020 by Singing Dragon,
an imprint of Jessica Kingsley Publishers
An Hachette Company

1

A CIP catalogue record for this title is available from the British Library and
the Library of Congress

ISBN 978 1 78775 628 1
eISBN 978 1 78775 631 1

Printed and bound in China by Leo Paper Products

Jessica Kingsley Publishers' policy is to use papers that are natural, renewable
and recyclable products and made from wood grown in sustainable forests.
The logging and manufacturing processes are expected to conform to the
environmental regulations of the country of origin.

Jessica Kingsley Publishers
73 Collier Street
London N1 9BE, UK

www.singingdragon.com

Dedicated to Bob and Be Insley

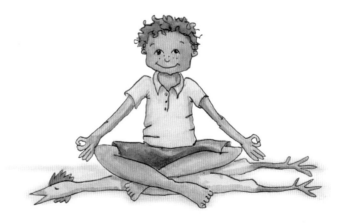

Acknowledgements

I would like to thank the following people for their honesty, encouragement and book enhancing suggestions: Sarah Peacock, Angela Tuck, David Morris, Jan Downey, Beth Whitehouse, Michelle Mathews, Lindsey Walsh, Evelyn Pope, Mandy Perry and the boys and girls of the Downfield Primary School Choir, Cheshunt, Hertfordshire.

Contents

INTRODUCTION

Thank you. Today you have shown that you *are* and certainly *will be* a superb children's yoga teacher.

Yes, today *you* are the one person in the yoga and educational world who is bothering to read this introduction. The rest of them have gone straight to the heart of the book – *The Games*. The rest of them are busy thumbing the contents looking for a game that will steal the show in front of a cynical headteacher, or grab the attention of a fidgety, feisty, bored Year 6 (5th grade) class, or be the magic bullet to taming the 'Reception (or pre-kindergarten) class from hell'.

So thank you for your time and well done. You will be the only person who understands not only *which* games to play, but also *which part of the lesson to play them in*. You will be the only teacher whose classroom management skills will shine, shine, shine, because you will have learnt how to structure your yoga lessons simply and effectively. You will have finished your planning and preparation and will be enjoying yourself. Your professionalism will be praised to the rafters. You will be in demand.

This is the book that I wished that *I* had had when I was starting out – a book that would have been my bible for my day-to-day teaching. My book will show you WHAT to teach, WHEN to teach it and HOW to teach it. This book will save you hours of planning and rummaging for resources and provide you with yoga games that the children will love.

Within these pages I have distilled 20 years of my work as a specialist children's yoga teacher. It is the perfect guide to teaching yoga to children as part of the curriculum or school day. And even though I have fought ferociously against after school and breakfast yoga clubs, and the now trendy family yoga classes, ironically, this book will be an enormous asset even in those situations.

Above all I wrote it to help you make sure that ALL children who you teach are included in the yoga lesson regardless of impairment, need, culture, shape, mood or size; and I have structured it so that you can get going immediately.

WHO THIS BOOK IS FOR

This book is for primary and elementary school teachers, special needs teachers, teaching assistants, nursery teachers, early years specialists, headteachers. In fact, everyone and anyone who works with children. It is also for parents who want to teach yoga to their children.

Of course, it is also for specialist children's yoga teachers.

Clearly written for folk in education who have little or no knowledge of yoga, as well as yoga folk who do, it shows that the key to a successful lesson is:

- structure,
- engagement,
- classroom management…
- and the yoga – *in that order.*

That said, the more you know, the better a teacher you will become, so if you do not have much yoga knowledge and understanding I hope this kickstarts a deeper interest in yoga.

WHO THIS BOOK IS *NOT* FOR

This book is definitely *not* for people who need to read step-by-step instructions on how to do yoga postures. I have made it easy. Just look at the pictures of the postures. That will show you what to do. Even better, show them to the children and they will see what they need to do. That's a promise. At this level we are not looking for perfection.

Neither is this book for people who wish to include those aspects of yoga that carry a mystical or spiritual label. Aspects like chanting 'om' and 'chakras' do not, in my opinion, have a place in children's yoga.

Finally, this book is not for folk who turn up without a lesson plan or an inkling of classroom management skills, who believe that they can 'sense' the needs of the students in front of them. As if!

THE HEART OF THIS BOOK

The two basic principles

At the heart of my teaching are *two* basic principles:

1   Children's yoga is most vibrant and has the greatest positive impact when taught as part of the integrated school curriculum. That means that it needs to be timetabled

weekly. For example as part of the physical education (PE) and personal, social and health education (PSHE) curriculum.

2   The best approach is a games approach. I find that pupils are eagerly engaged with the games approach – more so than *any other* approach. The core reasons are that:
  ◆ yoga games are fun
  ◆ learning outcomes are easier to achieve
  ◆ classroom management is more manageable.

I honestly believe that the children I have taught have learnt more social skills, have become better listeners, have grasped how to resolve disputes and have become more assertive through my yoga games. For my part it has been easier to formulate and achieve learning outcomes using the games approach.

It follows, therefore, that the methods, strategies and teaching approaches offered in the book are based on children's yoga lessons that are part of the regular weekly timetable; are delivered between 9.00am and 3.00pm; are practised in the school hall (or gymnasium); involve whole classes, i.e. 25 to 33 children; will have another adult in attendance (either the class teacher or teaching assistant or often both); where each child is assured of her own mat; and that the mats are set in a large circle.

STRUCTURE OF THE LESSON

When I am teaching I am highly structured. That does not mean that I am rigid or inflexible. Far from it, in fact, in my mind I am working in a gigantic aircraft hangar in which my structure allows me to:
  ◆ capitalise on learning opportunities
  ◆ capitalise on opportunities to help raise a child's self-esteem
  ◆ achieve my learning objectives
  ◆ teach with pace
  ◆ effectively manage the class and any behaviours that are presented to me.

My lessons are structured into SEVEN simple stages:
1   beginning
2   sequence
3   development
4   calming
5   relaxation
6   plenary
7   ending and exit.

For each stage you can choose a game that will achieve whatever you are trying to achieve. It is as simple as that. For example, in the development stage, you may be focusing on improving balancing and teamwork skills. *Brilliant Balancers* would target both learning objectives. And if you are only targeting balancing skills, then improved teamwork is a bonus.

Here is a little more about each stage, with examples of games best suited for that stage. Have a look at the chart on page 14 that shows the structure of the lesson with examples of games and an idea of timing.

Beginning

I expect the class to come in quietly, to take off shoes, socks and sweatshirts and put them away tidily on a bench or space that I have prepared. Ideally the class teacher will have organised this before they get to the hall, but that rarely happens.

I also expect every child to find a mat and sit down quietly in *Good Sitting Posture* waiting quietly for me to begin the lesson. Set the tone for the lesson as early as possible and you are off to a great start.

Depending on the year group you can then play a game like *Knock Down the Tower* or *Sitting on a Chicken*, which helps to improve posture. Or perhaps the *Banana Game*, which is about concentration and listening skills, as well as a terrific warm-up. Incidentally all three games involve a competitive element of class versus teacher, which most children love.

Sequence

I will talk later in more detail about the importance of sequences in the children's yoga lesson. During the sequence I encourage every pupil to join in, to concentrate and to perform the sequence as a class. I also encourage children to lead the class in a responsible and exemplary way.

A whole class practising *Sun Sequence* in the hall on a circle of mats brings the class together in a way like no other.

Development

This is the main activity or main game. The children love games like *Mixing Game*, *Rock Paper Scissors* and *Brilliant Balancers*. All the games in this book will help to improve listening, cooperation, teamwork and a host of social skills.

Calming

The development stage is normally a fun, often frantic and generally noisy time, so this stage has the purpose of calming pupils (students) in readiness for relaxation. It also helps bring any children who are 'on the ceiling' back to normality and is excellent for overall control of the class. Invariably I will use the *Rainstick Game* at this stage, when I expect pupils to be in *Good Sitting Posture* with their eyes gently closed listening out for the wonderful soothing sound of the rainstick.

Relaxation

There can be little argument that relaxation is beneficial for children, whether at school or at home. Changing from the calming stage to relaxation I expect pupils to move quietly showing respect for other pupils' space and their right to be still, calm and relaxed without interference.

Invariably I will use the *Ladybird Relaxation*, which has been the jewel in the crown of my yoga lessons for nearly two decades (Chissick and Peacock 2013) when I expect the children to be as still as possible in the supine position (lying on backs) on their own mat.

Plenary

With relaxation over we come into the plenary stage. By now the children are usually very relaxed, happy and secure. This stage is an ideal opportunity to ask for whole-class feedback, for example: 'Hands up if you enjoyed your yoga lesson'.

You can ask individual children: What did you enjoy best? Or you could reinforce a teaching point or posture, or find out who achieved their learning objective, or find out if activities work, and if children have understood a concept.

In addition you could use this stage to praise specific pupils for genuine improvements, not only in posture work, but also perhaps, in their behaviour. I often encourage pupils to compliment classmates on specific achievements. There is nothing more powerful than peers and teachers combining and focusing honest praise on a pupil.

Ending and exit

I expect pupils to leave calmly, quietly and relaxed, being in the right frame of mind for the next lesson on their timetable. All the good work of the previous 28 minutes can be wasted if you dare to neglect this stage. Best to devise a strategy that helps you achieve the quiet, thoughtful exit.

I have several – the most successful being when I ask the class to curl down in *Sleeping Bird Posture*.

I ask the children to stay in posture until they are
tapped on the shoulder. That is the signal to stand
up and line up quietly by the door. The posture
is seen very much as an introverted, quietening
posture that does the job admirably. Also, if there

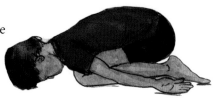

are any rewards on offer, such as stickers or certificates, I tend to leave them to
the very last moment before departure. It is a dangling carrot that has always worked
well for me and invariably means a quiet transition from yoga to their next lesson

STRUCTURE OF THE LESSON WITH EXAMPLES OF GAMES AND TIMING.

STAGE	ACTIVITY	EXAMPLES	TIMING (MINUTES)
Beginning	Coming in quietly Encourage good sitting and concentration	Good Sitting Banana Game	4
Sequence	Sequence	Sun Game Sun Sequence Yoga Detective What's Missing?	4
Development	Game or Main Activity	Umbrella Game Hoop Game Shark Game Sneaky Trees	7
Calming	Calming Activities	Rain Stick	4
Relaxation	Relaxation	Ladybird Relaxation	5
Plenary	Opportunities for feedback, for praise, to reinforce a teaching point or posture, to find out if activities work, if children understand a concept	Who helped you? Compliment time What new thing did you learn today? What did you like best? What went well for you?	4
Ending and Exit	Leaving calmly and quietly, being in right frame of mind for the next lesson	Sleeping Bird Shoes and socks on Lining up Presentation of reward	2

USING A VISUAL TIMETABLE

A visual timetable is a key structure in my yoga lessons. I would not dream of teaching
a lesson without one. It is imperative – a must have. If I were assessing a student

teacher who turned up without a visual timetable I would fail them on the spot. That is how strongly I feel.

The what and when of the lesson

The idea is simple: children can see *what* they will be doing and *when* they will be doing it. This is particularly important for children on the autistic spectrum, because 'it provides a structure and creates predictability, something that children with autism crave' (Sutton 2013).

Here's mine

Here are pictures of the stand that holds my visual timetable.

I tend to position the stand in the same place each time, normally where everyone can see it as they enter the hall.

It was originally designed as a magazine or leaflet display stand, but I have adjusted it to suit my purposes admirably. It folds down into a small bag so it is easy to carry into school, but the greatest benefit is that, when set up, it is lightweight and easy to move about the hall. This means that I can put it wherever the situation dictates.

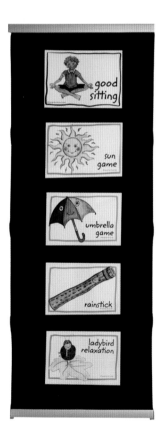
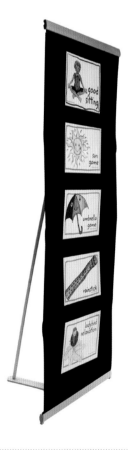

With nursery class

For example, when the nursery class (kindergarten) line up in readiness to leave the hall, I bring the stand over to *them*. I choose three or four children to come out individually to point to the posture card on the stand that they liked best. They can tell the class in their loudest voice what they liked best, for example, 'I liked *Sun Game*'. This is good practice in speaking skills and is often the opportunity for shyer children to gain some confidence.

Versatility

I have many examples that illustrate the benefits of the movability of the stand. 'Tania' is a six-year-old (Year 1) child from Russia who suffers from cerebral palsy. This makes moving around difficult without her walking frame. I move the timetable to her so that she can point out her favourite posture and practise her English at the same time.

Posture cards

Typically my timetable consists of posture cards, which show which postures we will be doing, and game cards, which show which games are to be played. Here are some examples of my posture and games cards.

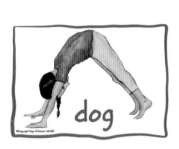 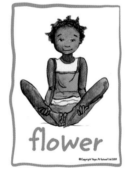 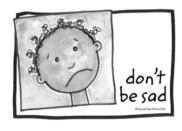

Pupils can clearly identify which postures and games make up the lesson and the running order.

Benefits

When a visual timetable is a regular part of the lesson there are many benefits. For example, it sends out a clear message to your pupils and other teaching staff that you have planned the lesson, that there is, indeed, structure, and that you are professional and know what you are doing.

There have been several occasions when classes have arrived earlier than scheduled after the break (recess), or I have been delayed. Invariably I would arrive in the hall to find the whole class waiting for me quietly in *Good Sitting Posture*. Why? Because they can take their direction from the visual timetable and they know what my expectations are in terms of their behaviour and attitude.

The silent lesson

Often towards the end of each half term I teach a 'silent' lesson when I do not speak at all. I greet the class with a card that says 'Hello' and end with a card that says 'Goodbye!'

Throughout the lesson I control and guide the class using the posture and game cards on the visual timetable. Of course, I also use a variety of facial expressions, body language and whatever it takes, but I DO NOT TALK!

This approach works well for six reasons:

1   The visual timetable has been central to the previous lessons.
2   I have only to point at the posture or game card and the children understand what to do.
3   I have kept to the same content and learning objectives for the previous four weeks.
4   By lesson five the class have learnt and can perform the postures and sequences with confidence.
5   The children feel secure because they are familiar with the structure.
6   The children know what I expect of them in terms of effort and behaviour.

Keeping track and getting stuck

Teaching seven to eight classes a day it is easy to lose track. The visual timetable helps *me* to keep my eye on the ball. Over the years I have experimented with different ways to display the timetable. At one time I was using a six-foot wooden plank that had a strip of Velcro down the centre.

One day I was teaching at a special needs school with low ceilings. As I walked into a classroom the plank wedged itself between the floor and ceiling. Of course I carried on regardless. Later, thanks to the caretaker's heavy mallet, the plank was set free and ceremoniously dumped in the nearest skip.

'John'

I will never forget 'John'. At the time he was a Key Stage 3 (aged between 11 and 14 years) pupil at a special needs school where I teach. He was one of a large group made up of three classes of children mainly with autism spectrum disorder (ASD). John was a big fella and his movement slow and cumbersome. Every week he would lumber in, look around and, after much coaxing, sit in *Good Sitting Posture*. I was never sure if he was truly engaged or even happy to be in yoga. One day, in my haste I transposed two posture cards thereby changing the order on the timetable. John became extremely upset, would not sit on a mat, charged around and eventually came over to the visual timetable to point at my mistake. I simply changed their positions and John was himself again. I learnt TWO important lessons from that:

1   Never underestimate the power of a visual timetable when teaching children with special needs – especially children with ASD.
2   Always assume that children are interacting with the visual timetable, 'even if it doesn't seem as if they are' (Delaney 2009). Apply this maxim to ALL children but especially to those with sensory and neurological impairments.

AIMS, OBJECTIVES AND OUTCOMES

Having clear aims and learning objectives or outcomes is essential and is part of the structure of the lesson.

My aims

Whichever age of children I am teaching, there are specific skills and target areas that form the general aims that run throughout my teaching approach. I do not need to include them in every lesson plan because they are embedded in my approach and are second nature to me now. They are based on teaching and improving or enhancing the following skills and aspects:

- self-control
- self-esteem
- teamwork
- taking turns
- speaking
- working to a time limit
- waiting
- concentrating
- sharing
- following rules of the game
- listening
- social skills
- independence
- participating
- leading the class
- looking
- decision-making
- being assertive.

In addition to that, and more aimed at special needs and nursery (kindergarten) children:

- anticipating what comes next
- finishing number sequences, posture sequences and lines to songs.

Specific learning outcomes

Whether you prefer to use the term learning objective or learning outcome is up to you. It is a fiercely contested debate among both educators and yoga teachers. I am more comfortable with *outcomes* because it implies that I can assess or measure achievement and also because it sounds better and suits my teaching style.

There are many ways to formulate learning outcomes. I have learnt many over the years both from my experience as a primary (elementary) school teacher and a yoga teacher. I have also had to *unlearn* many too. It is pointless overburdening yourself and the children with too many learning outcomes. At the very least if you have those aims that I have outlined above embedded in your approach you will win.

Recently a young man came to me for training. He teaches PE and looks after the entire physical activities programme at a special needs school in the Midlands. He reminded me that yoga and other physical activities are often the only place in the school day where some children can achieve something tangible without the pressure of obtaining a target or level rating. Reaching targets or levels in the curriculum and the pressure that imposes upon teachers and pupils is, as I write, unprecedented.

I do not grade or give a child a level of achievement in yoga either in terms of posture or social skill. Simply, they are encouraged to do their best and improve in both. If a child has learnt to relax using my legendary *Ladybird Relaxation* I do not feel a need to move that child up to 'a next stage'. Is it not enough and wonderful that he has the skill and knowledge to relax? For heaven's sake, do we want him to be working towards a PhD in relaxation?

That said, whether you teach yoga to children in schools or the community, it is essential that you are clear about your learning outcomes. You must have a lesson plan, and better still a scheme of work that helps you achieve your learning outcomes and shows progression in your planning.

Over the years I have got into the habit of sharing learning outcomes with the class when I felt it was appropriate. For example, one of the main learning objectives of *Rock Paper Scissors* game is: 'Can I disagree with others without getting angry?'

You need to make the learning outcome clear to the class before you start and ensure, as best you can, that most pupils grasp *what* they are trying to achieve and *how* they will achieve it.

I show specific learning outcomes for each game. For example in *Rock Paper Scissors* as follows:

LEARNING OUTCOMES
> Can I perform *Dragonfly*, *Tiger* and *Flamingo Postures* as part of a group?
> Can I disagree with others without getting angry?

You will notice that I have framed the outcomes in the form of a question. I do this for two educationally sound reasons:

1 Children can self-assess during and at the completion of the task.
2 Some children may be intimidated by an outcome that is framed as 'I can…' because they may believe that *they cannot*.

ENOUGH ALREADY WITH THE GUIDANCE – LET THE GAMES BEGIN!

REFERENCES

Chissick, M. and Peacock, P. (2013) *Ladybird's Remarkable Relaxation: How Children (and Frogs, Dogs, Flamingos and Dragons) Can Use Yoga Relaxation to Help Deal with Stress, Grief, Bullying and Lack of Confidence.* London: Jessica Kingsley Publishers.

Delaney, T. (2009) *101 Games and Activities for Children with Autism, Asperger's and Sensory Processing Disorders.* New York: McGraw-Hill.

Sutton, T. (2013) 'Visual timetables', *Special Children*, Issue 216.

THE GAMES

THE WHAT, WHEN AND HOW OF CHILDREN'S YOGA

The WHAT is about choosing the game
that matches the learning objectives
that you want to achieve.

The WHEN is about fitting it into the
relevant stage of the lesson.

The HOW is simply teaching the game
as it appears in this book.

BEGINNING GAMES

GOOD SITTING GAME

There is a lot going on with this simple starting game. It grabs attention, encourages immediate movement, which is a good up-stretch, it's easy to follow and offers the contrast of silence and sound. It's great fun, especially if you add the ingredient of trying to catch out pupils and adults.

AGE: 3–7 years (Nursery–Year 2)
POSTURES: Good Sitting
SKILLS: Focusing, self-control
RESOURCES: Posture and Game card

LEARNING OUTCOMES
❯ Can I sit quietly in *Good Sitting* with straight back and my fingers and thumbs touching?

What to do
Have the children in *Good Sitting Posture*. Stretch your arms above your head saying or singing 'Good Sitting'. Encourage the class to follow or copy you. Bring your arms down and sit quietly in *Good Sitting,* counting up to five obviously and quietly. Repeat twice more, lengthening the time sitting quietly to a count of ten. Try to catch out children and adults by bluffing that you are about to stretch up and say 'Good Sitting'.

The game becomes a battle of wits…will you stretch up or will you not?

SITTING ON A CHICKEN

Children cheer when they know the *Chicken Game* is on the timetable. Ideally played at the beginning of the lesson, it will encourage straight backs and quiet focusing, as well as setting the tone for the lesson in terms of class management and behaviour expectation. It is one of those games of 'them versus you', which children love – especially when you lose.

AGE: 7–11 years (Year 3–Year 6)
POSTURES: Good Sitting
SKILLS: Focusing, self-control
RESOURCES: 3 × small laminated chicken cards – see Resources page 91

LEARNING OUTCOMES

❯ Can I sit quietly in *Good Sitting* with straight back and my fingers and thumbs touching?

What to do

The children are on mats in *Good Sitting Posture*.

Ask another adult to find three children who deserve to be sitting on a chicken card by virtue of:

◆ straight backs
◆ quiet focus
◆ thumb and index finger touching
◆ warm friendly smile.

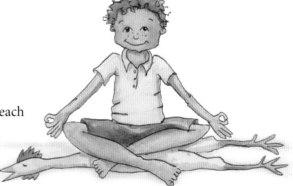

Your adult helper gives the chosen three each a small laminated chicken card. While this is happening you are 'hiding your eyes'.

Your task is then to return to the circle to guess who is sitting on a chicken.

What can happen?

The older the year group the more they will try to bluff, for example by *not* smiling, which is great fun, yet in a quiet way.

BANANA GAME

Such a simple game, yet an *all time favourite* because the children love *not* being caught out by teacher. This is also a great warm-up activity.

AGE: 3–7 years (Nursery–Year 2)
POSTURES: Banana
SKILLS: Listening, participating, following rules of the game
RESOURCES: The occasional banana

LEARNING OUTCOMES

> Can I make a banana shape with my arms and body?
> Can I stop when my teacher stops?
> Can I hold the posture quietly?

What to do

Children stand on their mats (or in front of their chairs) in *Stick Posture.*
Teacher demonstrates *Banana Posture* and sings the banana song:

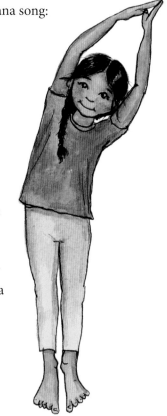

> *I'm a banana*
> *I'm a banana*
> *I'm a banana, nana, nana, nana*
> *I'm a banana*
> *Oh I'm a banana*
> *I'm a banana, nana, nana*
> *Nooh*

When the children are familiar with the posture and the song, explain that you have a target of (say) four children who will be caught out if they continue to sing or move when you have stopped, i.e. children are to hold the posture in silence where they stop. Most children will try hard not to be caught out. This wonderful side stretch is a terrific warm-up. The song is very catchy too.

Extensions

As the children become more accustomed to the game, increase your target figure.

KNOCK DOWN THE TOWER GAME

This is a wonderful way to engage the class immediately, especially for the first time. Everyone will want to be picked. You will be spoilt for choice. Who doesn't want to knock down the tower? They will be eating out of your hand.

AGE: 4–8 years (Reception, Year 1–Year 3)
POSTURES: Good Sitting
SKILLS: Listening, following instructions, self control
RESOURCES: Foam blocks to build tower

LEARNING OUTCOMES

❯ Can I sit quietly in *Good Sitting* with straight back and my fingers and thumbs touching?

What to do

Build a tower of colourful foam bricks in the middle of the hall. Best to do this before children come in because of the element of surprise. Ask the class who would like to knock the tower down. You will be inundated. Tell the class that you will choose someone sitting well in *Good Sitting Posture*.

Make your choice. Give the pupil the choice of knocking down the tower calmly or angrily. This may be something you can refer to later.

BEAT THE CLOCK

Children love to start the lesson with this game. They enjoy the healthy competiveness of trying to beat their own score going quickly from *Good Sitting* to *Stick* and then back again. You'll find lots of opportunities to discuss tactics with the older children too.

AGE: 6–11 years (Year 2–Year 6)
POSTURES: Stick, Good Sitting
SKILLS: Participating, concentration, listening and following instructions
RESOURCES: Game card, stopwatch

LEARNING OUTCOMES

> Can I be alert in *Good Sitting/Stick*?
> Can I react quickly?
> Can I think of a tactic or way to be faster?
> Can I estimate time taken?

What to do

Everyone is in *Good Sitting* including you. You start the stopwatch, stand in *Stick* and call out someone's name. They in turn stand in *Stick* and call out someone's name, who in turn stands in *Stick*, and so on.

When the last person stands in *Stick*, you stop the stopwatch and check the time and announce it to the class.

Now reverse the activity. Start the stopwatch, sit down into *Good Sitting Posture* and call out someone's name. They in turn sit down into *Good Sitting* and call out someone's name, and so on. When the last person has sat down, stop the stopwatch and ask the class to guess which 'way' was quicker: *Good Sitting* to *Stick* or *Stick* to *Good Sitting*.

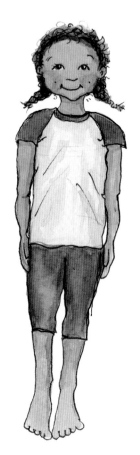

THE WRONG POSTURE

A simple game that involves and engages the whole class quickly and is brilliant for the early part of the yoga lesson.

AGE: 6–11 years (Year 2–Year 6)
POSTURES: Choose three contrasting postures, e.g. *Butterfly*, *Crab*, *Tree*
SKILLS: Concentration, listening and quick thinking
RESOURCES: Posture cards

LEARNING OUTCOMES
› Can I concentrate?
› Can I react quickly?
› Can I follow instructions?

What to do
Decide which three postures to use in the game. Set them out in a triangle for everyone to see.

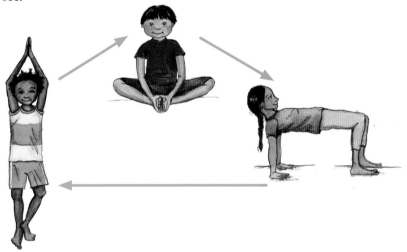

The idea is that when you say *Tree Posture*, for example, you want *all* the children to come into *Butterfly*, or whatever the next posture is going clockwise around the triangle.

It helps if you throw a ball to someone in the circle. It keeps them on their toes. Repeat several times.

You can change the order of postures or bring in new ones.

SEQUENCES

THE IMPORTANCE OF SEQUENCE IN THE YOGA LESSON

What is the Sun Sequence?

The *Sun Sequence*, also known as *Sun Salutation*, *Salute to the Sun* (*Surya Namaskar* to yoga buffs) is one of the most popular and integral parts of any yoga lesson – children's or adult's. Simply put, it is a series of flowing yoga postures.

What are the benefits?

One of the objectives of the sequence is to move the spine in a variety of ways to increase flexibility. If you have tried it you will know that it exercises the whole body. Some people use it as part of their wake up morning routine; others as a bedtime solution to help sleep. If you are short of time it can act as a whole session.

Apart from the fact that children love them, sequences are highly effective in children's lessons for several reasons:

- Children enjoy the security of the structure that sequences bring – they feel more secure knowing what is coming next.
- Sequences demand concentration and coordination.
- They provide opportunities for children to step up and lead the class.
- Children enjoy the flowing body movement.
- It is a more invigorating way to practise compared to isolated postures.
- Some children find sequences easy to remember and can teach them to friends and family members.

I have taught *Children's Sun Sequence* in every possible situation that you can imagine. That includes children with the most challenging and severe physical needs, children across the autistic spectrum, children with intense emotional and behavioural needs, Early Years children and the whole range of mainstream primary school-aged children.

INCLUSION, INCLUSION, INCLUSION

Over the years I have developed sequences that ensure that every child is included. I have grouped them into four basic sequences, which can be used in an appropriate situation to ensure that every child is included. They are:

1   *Sun Game* – which is a standing sequence for children of 3–6 years (Nursery, Reception and Year 1).
2   *Sun Sequence* – which is a standing sequence for mainstream primary children from the ages of 6–11 years (Year 2 to Year 6).
3   *Sun Game in Wheelchairs* – which is for children in wheelchairs.
4   *Sitting Sun Sequence* – which has been developed for children of 6–11 years who find it difficult to stand, e.g. those with cerebral palsy or with a temporary injury like a broken leg.

All four sequences have been tried, tested and developed in schools for nearly two decades – so you know they will work.

The age range that I suggest for each sequence is a sensible guide for you, but it's not set in stone. I encourage you to be flexible and use the appropriate sequence to match the needs of the children in front of you. For example, I was teaching a new class of 10–11 years olds (Year 6) recently in which there was a boy with cerebral palsy. It was appropriate to use Sun Game rather than Sun Sequence in order to make sure he was included. Of course I adjusted my teaching approach and vocabulary to meet the needs of the class of 10–11 year olds. The same principle would apply with Sun Game in Wheelchairs.

Pupils with Autism

I have also developed a sequence for children on the Autism Spectrum that I use specifically in Special Needs Schools and schools that specialise in ASD pupils. That is for another book. Nevertheless you will encounter an increasing number of children on the Autism Spectrum in mainstream schools and it is vital that you are able to ensure that they are included. The sequence stage of the lesson is the stage where you have the greatest opportunity in engaging ASD pupils because my sequences are:

◆   Simple
◆   Highly structured
◆   Easy to remember
◆   Easy to repeat

Furthermore, by repeating the same sequence week after week, session after session the ASD pupil will feel more secure knowing what is coming next and, in my experience, will engage.

'Taz'

'Taz' was 8 years old when he suddenly appeared in a Year 3 class a few weeks into the academic year. He was placed in mainstream education because he was waiting for a place in a special school. He had challenging, complex sensory, behavioural and communication needs and was non-verbal. Taz had a learning support assistant (LSA) with him for most of the school day. Taz would come into yoga with his LSA.

We had been practising *Sun Sequence* prior to three weeks before Taz's arrival. I realised immediately that *Sun Sequence* would be a step too far for Taz. So I switched to *Sun Game*. Taz's LSA helped him through each part of the sequence, literally moving him into the various postures. It was not easy because he was a big boy. Nevertheless we all persevered and, little by little, week-by-week Taz did more of the *Sun Game* independently.

Eventually, by the end of the summer term he actually led the class in *Sun Game*, albeit without speaking. We adults wept tears of happiness and the whole class clapped their hands red.

Taz is an extreme example. However, I have taught countless ASD children with a range of abilities in mainstream who thrived in the sequence section because of the structure, simplicity and repetition.

1. SUN GAME

Simple, easy to learn and fun, and serves as a foundation for the more challenging sequence in later years.

AGE: 3–6 years (Nursery, Reception and Year 1)
POSTURES: As shown in diagram
SKILLS: Sequencing, leading, listening
RESOURCES: Game card

LEARNING OUTCOMES

> Can I follow instructions?
> Can I remember what comes next in Sun Game?
> Can I be the Teacher in Sun Game?

What to do

Learn and practise the *Sun Sequence*.

You lead the sequence by calling out the individual elements of the sequence in the order shown on the chart while performing that posture. The children, as a class, call them back to you while performing the posture too.

For example, you say 'Stick' as you come into *Stick Posture*. The children call 'Stick' back to you as they too come into *Stick Posture*…and so on.

You can slow or quicken the pace, increase or lower the volume of your voice, even lead in silence.

You can increase the time held in each posture to match the needs and abilities of the class.

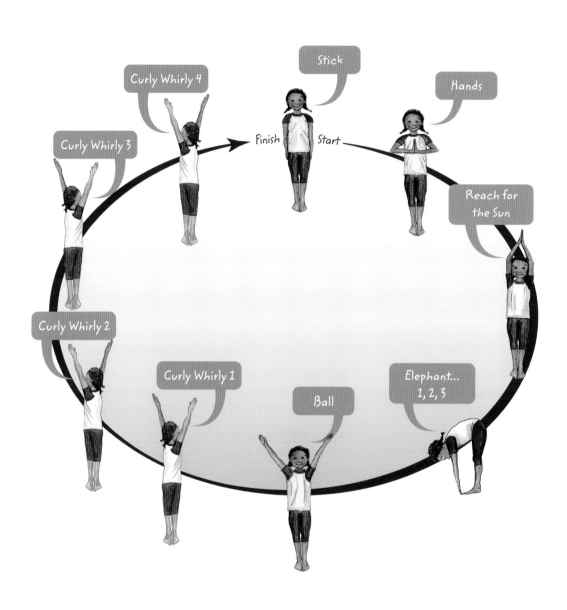

2. SUN SEQUENCE

This sequence has been developed for older children, is more challenging than the Sun Game and includes more postures.

AGE: 6–11 years (Year 2–Year 6)
POSTURES: As shown in diagram
SKILLS: Sequencing, leading, listening and following instructions
RESOURCES: Game card

LEARNING OUTCOMES

› Can I remember the order of postures in Sun Sequence?
› Can I perform each posture?
› Can I lead my class in Sun Sequence?
› Can I teach my friends and Family Sun Sequence?
› Can I identify the benefits of Sun Sequence?

What to do

You lead the sequence by calling out the individual elements of the sequence in the order shown on the chart while performing that posture. The children, as a class, call them back to you while performing the posture too.

For example, you say 'Stick' as you come into *Stick Posture*. The children call 'Stick' back to you as they too come into *Stick Posture*…and so on.

You can slow or quicken the pace, increase or lower the volume of your voice, even lead in silence.

You can increase the time held in each posture to match the needs and abilities of the class.

There are a host of games based on *Sun Sequence*. *Sun Sequence* is a terrific warm-up activity.

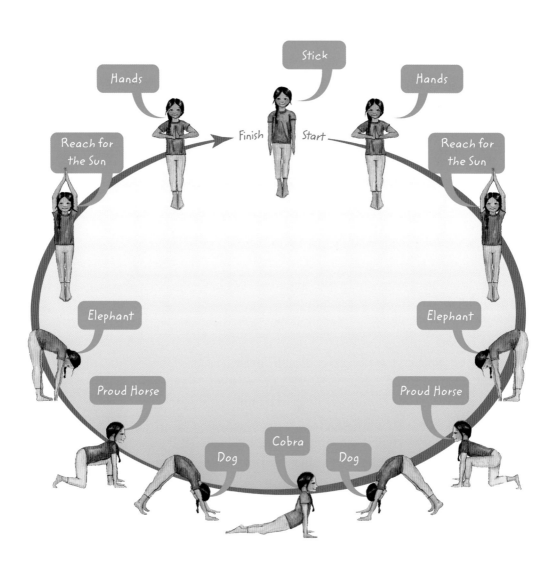

3. SUN GAME IN WHEELCHAIRS

I love this sequence because children in wheelchairs are immediately involved with their classmates, with everyone in the same posture together.

AGE: 6–11 years (Year 2–Year 6)
POSTURES: As shown in diagram
SKILLS: Listening, sequencing, leading and following instructions
RESOURCES: Game card

LEARNING OUTCOMES

> Can I remember the order of postures?
> Can I perform each posture?
> Can I lead my class in Sun Game?
> Can I teach my friends and Family Sun Game?
> Can I identify the benefits of Sun Game?

What to do

Learn and practise this sequence. Make sure the child (or children) in the wheelchair is part of the circle of mats.

You lead by calling out the individual elements of the sequence in the order shown on the chart while performing that posture. The children, as a class, call them back to you while performing the posture too

For example: You say 'Stick ' as you come into *Stick* Posture. The children call 'Stick' back to you as they too come into 'Stick'… and so on.

You can slow or quicken the pace, increase or lower the volume of your voice, even lead in silence.

You can increase the time held in each posture to match the needs and abilities of the class.

Valuable Teaching Tip: I suggest you teach *Sun Game* rather the *Sun Sequence* regardless of the year group.

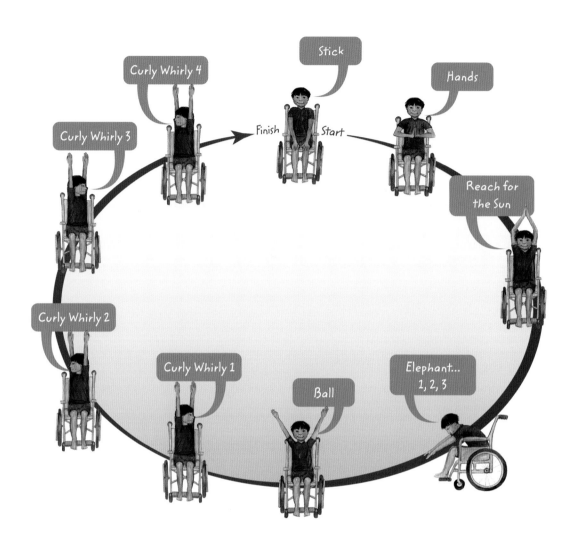

YOGA GAMES TO TEACH IN SCHOOLS

4. SITTING SUN SEQUENCE

This sequence was developed for children who have difficulty standing, but who still want to be challenged and like physical activity. For example it will be ideal for children with Cerebral Palsy. I also use it if someone has an injury, which prevents him or her from standing.

AGE: 6–11 Years (Year 2–Year 6)
POSTURES: As shown in diagram
SKILLS: Sequencing, leading, listening and following instructions
RESOURCES: Game card

LEARNING OUTCOMES

> Can I remember the order of postures in Sitting Sun Sequence?
> Can I remember which way to point my knees and nose in Curly Whirly posture?
> Can I identify the postures that are different to Sun Sequence?
> Can I lead my class in Sitting Sun Sequence?

What to do

Learn and practise the Sitting Sun Sequence.

You lead by calling out the individual elements of the sequence in the order shown on the chart while performing that posture. As a class, the children call them back to you while performing the posture too.

For example: You say 'Stick' as you come into Stick posture. The children call 'Stick' back to you as they come into 'Stick' and so on.

You can slow or quicken the pace, increase or lower the volume of your voice, even lead in silence.

You can increase the time held in each posture to match the needs and abilities of the class.

Valuable Teaching Tip: You can also use it as a change of routine to Sun Sequence because it presents a different set of postures and challenges to the children.

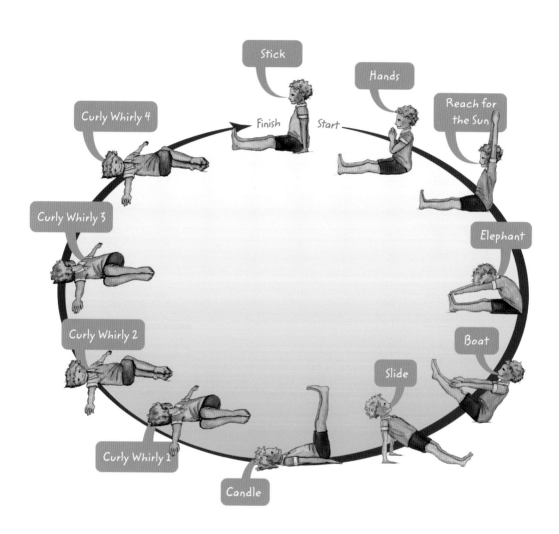

SEQUENCE GAMES

Having learnt the relative *Sun Sequence*, a great way to reinforce the benefits is to bring Sequence Games into your lesson plan. Here are six examples that children enjoy.

CHASE THE FROG

This game will keep pupils on their toes aware that at any moment they could be asked to lead. I call it *Chase the Frog* because I use a frog-shaped yoga block, but you can use anything – even a sponge. So…chase the sponge, shoe, smelly sock…

AGE: 6–11 years (Year 2–Year 6)
SUITABLE SEQUENCES: Sun Sequence, Sun Game in Wheelchair, Sitting Sun Sequence
SKILLS: Sequencing, concentration
RESOURCES: Foam frog, shoe, trainer, bean bag

LEARNING OUTCOMES
> Do I know what comes next in *Sun Sequence*?
> Am I alert?

What to do
Perform a round of *Sun Sequence* to reinforce the activity.

On the next round place the frog at the feet of a pupil.

That child becomes the leader, until you pick up the frog and place it at the feet of another child, who takes over from the previous child at the correct place in the sequence.

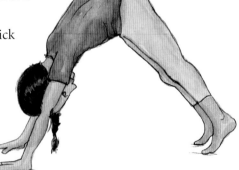

Continue to the end of the sequence and repeat.

YOGA DETECTIVE WHAT'S MISSING?

A wonderful game to reinforce and practise *Sun Sequence*. It is also a great opportunity to encourage shyer pupils to speak out in class.

AGE: 6–11 years (Year 2–Year 6)
SUITABLE SEQUENCES: Sun Game, Sun Sequence, Sun Game in Wheelchair, Sitting Sun Sequence
SKILLS: Sequencing, concentration
RESOURCES: Game card

LEARNING OUTCOMES
> Can I identify the missing part to the sequence?

What to do
Tell the class that:

1 You will lead the sequence and will leave out one part of the sequence.
2 You will decide which one to leave out before you start.
3 Their job as detectives is to spot which posture is missing.
4 They have to wait till the sequence is completed before offering their answers.

Call out the postures for the sequence, leaving out the *one* posture. When you've finished choose three 'yoga detectives' to say what is missing. Repeat once more.

Extensions
◆ Ask for a volunteer to lead. Remind them they need to decide which posture they will leave out of the sequence *before* starting.
◆ Miss out two, three or more parts of the sequence.
◆ Ask the detective to demonstrate the missing posture instead of saying it.

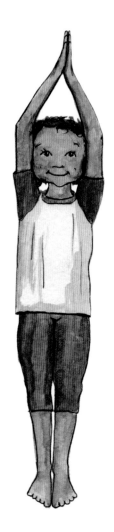

YOGA DETECTIVE WHO'S THE LEADER?

Like the other *Yoga Detective Games*, this is a wonderful game to reinforce and practise *Sun Sequence*. This activity helps children to focus on the detail.

AGE: 6–11 years (Year 2–Year 6)
SUITABLE SEQUENCES: Sun Sequence, Sun Game in Wheelchair, Sitting Sun Sequence
SKILLS: Sequencing, concentration
RESOURCES: Game card

LEARNING OUTCOMES
> Can I identify who is leading the sequence?
> Can I lead the sequence silently?

What to do
Choose a pupil to be the yoga detective and ask them to pop outside for a moment (or cover their eyes and ears). Choose another pupil to be the leader of the sequence and make sure that the rest of the class knows who the leader is. Call the detective back into the hall and ask them to stand in the centre of the circle and to rotate slowly as the class perform the *Sun Sequence*. Their task is to spot the leader.

The class takes their silent lead from the leader.

The detective has three guesses as to who the leader is.

Repeat the game only once more.

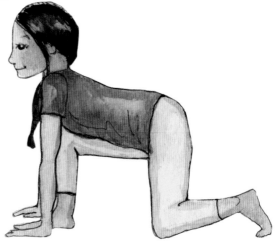

YOGA DETECTIVE WHO'S TALKING?

This is the funniest of the *Yoga Detective Games*. Children love it because it is an opportunity to disguise their voice, often with some outrageous results.

AGE: 8–11 years (Year 4–Year 6)
SUITABLE SEQUENCES: Sun Sequence, Sun Game in Wheelchair, Sitting Sun Sequence
SKILLS: Sequencing, concentration
RESOURCES: Game card

LEARNING OUTCOMES
› Can I identify who is leading the sequence by their voice?
› Can I lead the sequence in a disguised voice?

What to do
Choose a pupil to be the yoga detective and ask them to pop outside for a moment (or cover their eyes and ears).

Choose another pupil to be the leader of the sequence and make sure everyone knows who the leader is.

Ask the detective to return to the room and stand in the centre of the circle and have him or her blindfolded.

Emphasise the rule that the detective must slowly rotate as the rest of class perform the sequence. The class take their instructions from the leader starting and changing onto the next posture on his or her verbal instruction in the disguised voice.

The detective has three guesses as to the leader is.

Repeat once more.

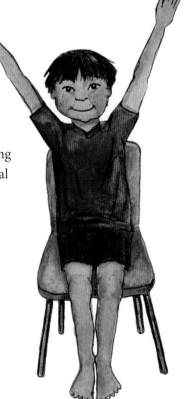

THE INCREDIBLE WEATHER GAME

Children love this game, especially in the summer when they will work to their best ability to be sprayed with water, cooled by the wind and shocked by the thunder.

AGE: 8–11 years (Year 4–Year 6)
SUITABLE SEQUENCES: Sun Sequence, Sun Game in Wheelchair, Sitting Sun Sequence
SKILLS: Sequencing, concentration
RESOURCES: Clean plastic plant spray bottle, large piece of foam or card, thunder tube or something that makes a thunder sound

LEARNING OUTCOMES

❯ Can I continue with a sequence even when it is hard to concentrate?

What to do

Lead the sequence. At an appropriate moment ask someone which weather they would like to choose from: wind, rain or thunder. If they choose rain, spray them with a fine spray of water; if they choose wind, use something big enough to flap cold wind onto them. If they choose thunder, I shake a special 'thunder tube' that I bought in a toyshop. You will find that the children will work hard to be chosen.

Continue with the sequence, stopping frequently to choose the next new 'victim'.

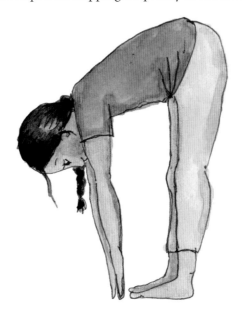

ONE BEHIND

This is a terrific concentration builder as well as one of those games where children love to rise to the bait that challenges their powers of concentration.

AGE: 8–11 years (Year 4–Year 6)
SUITABLE SEQUENCES: Sun Sequence, Sun Game in Wheelchair, Sitting Sun Sequence
SKILLS: Sequencing, concentration
RESOURCES: Game card

LEARNING OUTCOMES
❯ Can I completely concentrate on the sequence, even when the teacher tries to distract me?

What to do
Explain to the class that you will lead the sequence; that you will begin with *Stick*, upon which they will do and say nothing. Then, when you have said *Hands*, they come into *Stick*. When you say and come into *Reach for the Sun* they come into *Hands*. In other words they will be ONE BEHIND.

When it comes to the final instruction it is a good idea to say 'And nothing' or 'And blah blah' as their cue to say 'And Stick'.

Repeat.

You may want to ask one of the class to lead.

Extensions
1 Two Behind
2 Three Behind and, if you are very brave…
3 Four and Five Behind.

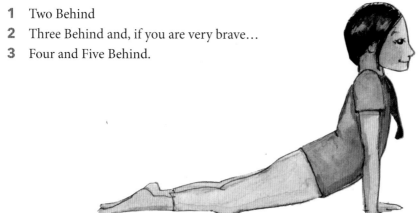

DEVELOPMENT GAMES

BRILLIANT BALANCERS

I was looking for a game which would help the children gain a better understanding that postures can be sorted into types or categories like, for example, balances, upside-down or side stretches, and which would also enable the children to learn the specific benefits of balancing. After weeks of tweaking *Brilliant Balancers* emerged and fulfilled all my criteria, and has become a great team game that the children love.

AGE: 6–11 years (Year 2–Year 6)
POSTURES: Tree, Flamingo, Boat, Tiger and Dancer
SKILLS: Balancing, concentration
RESOURCES: Game card and posture cards

LEARNING OUTCOMES

> Can I improve my teamwork skills?
> Can I improve my balancing postures?

What to do

Set up five or six mats at the centre of the circle as if they are the spokes of a wheel. Divide the class into five or six groups each containing five or six children. Allocate one of the five mats to each group. Have each group sit in *Good Sitting* and familiarise themselves with their team and the position of their mat.

Ask the children to return to a mat in the outer circle.

Explain that when you say 'NOW!' and name the posture, for example, *Flamingo*, the children need to get to their team mat quickly and get into the posture.

Explain also that you are looking for everyone in your team to be facing the same way and quietly focused. I award points to each group for achieving the goal.

Repeat at least five times to include all five postures.

BUTTERFLY SKITTLES

This game involves lots of exercise, determination and tactics as the children become butterfly skittles trying to stay in the game by avoiding the oncoming ball.

AGE: 8–11 years (Year 4–Year 6)
POSTURES: Butterfly, Chips
SKILLS: Concentration, tactics, thinking
RESOURCES: Game card, posture cards and 4 large sponge balls

LEARNING OUTCOMES

> Can I find a tactic to stay in the game?
> Can I improve my *Butterfly Posture*?

What to do

Introduce *Butterfly Posture* to the class.

Choose three children to be the 'ball rollers'. They position themselves around the hall. Assemble the rest of the class in the centre of the hall in *Butterfly Posture* facing outwards towards the 'ball rollers'.

The 'ball rollers' roll the balls towards the 'butterfly skittles' trying to get as many children out as possible. The children in *Butterfly* must stay in the posture; their task is to try their best to avoid the oncoming ball by rocking from side to side, back to front or any tactic they can think of…as long as they stay in posture.

When a butterfly is 'out', she stands in *Chips Posture* until the end of the game.

This game is fast and furious. It is best to stop after a few minutes and choose new ball rollers.

Repeat three times.

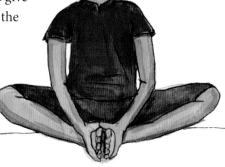

Valuable Teaching Tip: Choose four children to be 'ball getters'. Their job is to retrieve the balls and give them back to the ball rollers quickly. This keeps the game pacy.

Warning: They cannot get enough of this game!

CHIPS IN THE MUD

Chips in the Mud is a classic game, easy to teach, and is guaranteed to get children running around, thinking tactically and raise their heartbeat.

AGE: 6–11 years (Year 2–Year 6)
POSTURES: Chips
SKILLS: Concentration, listening, participating and thinking tactically
RESOURCES: Game card and posture card

LEARNING OUTCOMES
› Can I find a tactic to stay in the game?
› Can I improve my *Chips Posture*?

What to do
Choose two children to be 'the catchers'. They have to chase around and tag as many children as they can. When a child is tagged, they have to stand in *Chips Posture* as if stuck in the mud. The only way that they can be released is for a free person to crawl through their legs.

Continue for 3 minutes or until everybody is STUCK IN THE MUD!

Change the catchers and start again.

Extension
Increase the number of catchers.

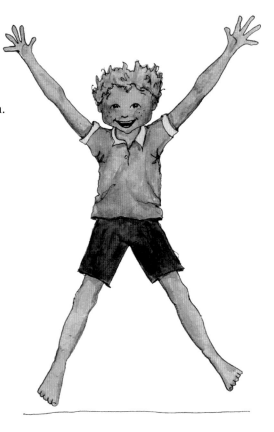

CONCENTRATION/MATCHING GAME – WHOLE CLASS

This is a fun, yet disciplined way to start the lesson. It builds on the famous memory game and is therefore demanding of concentration.

AGE: 7–11 years (Year 3–Year 6)
POSTURES: Various
SKILLS: Concentrating, observing, thinking, matching
RESOURCES: Five to six sets of posture cards

LEARNING OUTCOMES

> Can I improve my concentration?

What to do

Set up five or six pairs of posture cards at the centre of the circle. For example, you could use two boat postures, two dancer posture cards, and so on. At first, have them face-up so children can see what is there. Then turn them face-down and mix them up.

Choose individual children to try to match up two cards. Encourage the class to concentrate so as to pick out pairs. Obviously it may take a few goes. When someone matches two cards together the whole class performs that posture.

Continue for another two postures.

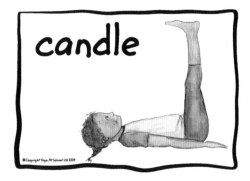 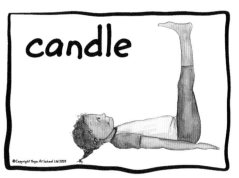

Valuable Teaching Tip: Play for a maximum of 4 minutes as a starter game.

CONCENTRATION/MATCHING GAME - IN SMALL GROUPS

Rather than playing with the whole class as in the previous game, there are lots of social skills to be worked on using this game in small groups.

AGE: 7–11 years (Year 3–Year 6)
POSTURES: Various
SKILLS: Cooperation, turn taking and rules of the game
RESOURCES: Five sets of matching game cards

LEARNING OUTCOMES

> Can I improve my concentration?
> Can I wait my turn?

What to do

Split the class into five or six groups each of five or six pupils. Each group sits in a small circle. Appoint a sensible person in each group to choose five sets of doubles and have them face-down within the circle. The object of the game is to match the posture cards. When a pair is matched the whole group performs the posture. Children will need to take turns and show consideration to each other. When all the pairs are matched, the game is over.

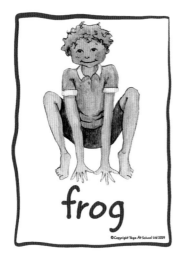
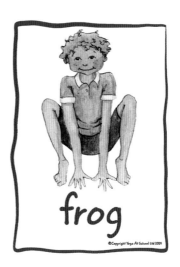

CROWN GAME

This is a fun way to reinforce postures. You can also introduce new ones as long as you are prepared for the children to tell you: 'We don't know this posture!' Plus it's a great activity to encourage speaking and listening skills.

AGE: 7–11 years (Year 3–Year 6)
POSTURES: Various
SKILLS: Thinking, listening and participating
RESOURCES: Adjustable crown, posture cards

LEARNING OUTCOMES
> Can I identify yoga postures?
> Can I work well in a group?

What to do
Make or buy a simple headband or crown upon which you can stick some Velcro.

Choose someone to wear the special headband or crown. Choose a posture card that is familiar to everyone and attach it using Velcro in a way so that the wearer cannot see it. The class performs the posture and the crown wearer tries to identify the posture.

If the guesser finds it difficult, then give them some clues until they guess the posture.

Choose a new guesser and a new posture and go again.

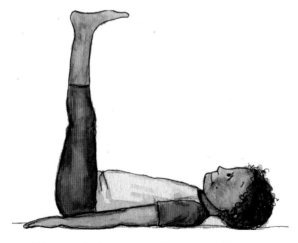

Valuable Teaching Tip: Works best in small groups where more people get to wear the crown and social skills can be worked on.

DOG RELAY

This game is brilliant for perseverance and teamwork. Also, because *Dog Posture* strengthens arms, legs and wrists and sends fresh blood to the head, children feel that they have had a jolly good workout.

AGE: 7–11 years (Year 3–Year 6)
POSTURES: Dog
SKILLS: Thinking, tactics and teamwork
RESOURCES: Game and posture cards

LEARNING OUTCOMES

> Can I work well with my team?
> Can I persevere with my task?

What to do

Divide the class into, say, three teams of around ten, or four teams of around seven, depending on your class. Place cones to show the starting line.

In each team everyone comes into *Dog Posture* forming a tunnel. Have the teams line up equally using the cones as a guide.

On the word 'GO', the team members at the back crawl through the tunnel to the front of the line and come into *Dog Posture*. When they are in position, the next person at the back then crawls through and comes into *Dog* at the front, and so on, until all team members have been through the tunnel.

The winning team sits in *Good Sitting* with their hands in the air.

Repeat three times.

Extension

Try this with *Chips Posture*.

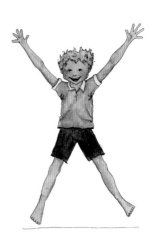

DON'T BE SAD

Here's a game to bring out everyone's acting skills and you get to teach five or six postures too. It can also trigger a little discussion on how postures (and exercise generally) can cheer you up when you are sad.

AGE: 3–7 years (Nursery, Reception–Year 2)
POSTURES: Various
SKILLS: Concentrating, following instructions, listening
RESOURCES: Game and posture cards

LEARNING OUTCOMES

> Can I listen well?
> Can I follow instructions?
> Can I remember the postures?

What to do

Tell the class that you are pretending to be sad. Stand at one end of the hall facing the class who are at the other end of the hall. They sing or say:

> Oh Michael, Oh Michael
> Don't be so sad.
> What shall we do
> To make you feel glad?

You reply, for example, take three steps sideways and come into *Tree Posture*.

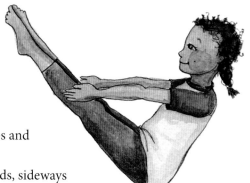

Continue, each time changing the posture and varying the number of steps and directions for them to take.

For example, send the class backwards, sideways or a mixture of all. The first child to touch you on the shoulder becomes the next sad person and the game starts again.

Extension

Replace 'sad' with 'grumpy' or 'angry'. You will need to change the lines too.

FLOWER GAME

A game that will plant the seeds of assertiveness when children hear their own strong voices saying: 'that's my view' or 'that's my opinion', while you model how to respect their view. Pretty soon early seeds of self-respect emerge inside and outside the yoga lesson. On top of that you all get to practise three popular postures.

AGE: 5–11 years (Year 1–Year 6)
POSTURES: Flower, Frog, Dog, Crab
SKILLS: Being assertive, concentrating, following instructions
RESOURCES: Game and posture cards

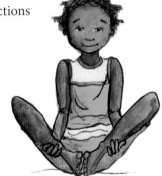

LEARNING OUTCOMES

> Can I perform *Flower/Crab/Frog/Dog Postures*?
> Can I travel in *Crab/Frog/Dog Postures*?
> Do I have good listening skills?
> Can I make my own decisions?

What to do

Teach the *Flower Posture*. Then teach *Crab*, *Dog* and *Frog* with movement. For example, *Moving Crab, Hopping Frog, Walking Dog*.

Choose three children to be the three 'listening flowers' who sit on blocks in the centre of your large circle.

'Listening flowers' sit in *Flower Posture* with their eyes closed and promise to keep them closed until you say open them.

Hold up *one* of three posture cards. Depending upon the posture you show, children cross the circle moving in the posture you have chosen, e.g. *Hopping Frog*.

After a while ask the children to return to a mat, come out of posture and be in *Good Sitting*. Ask the three 'flowers' to open their eyes.

Ask Flower 1: 'Which posture did we practise just now?' Encourage and model the difference between a question and a firm statement by reinforce with 'you asking me or telling me?'

If any flower says the same as another flower ask them if they are copying the other person. Model and encourage the flower to say 'That's my view, Michael' or 'That is my opinion, Mrs Jones'. Test the flower by urging him to change his mind.

Repeat with two other flowers.

Ask the class to show which posture they just did.

Repeat three times and change listening flowers.

FLEEING FROG

Any game that involves *Frog Posture* is good news for legs, knees, ankles and toes. This Frog Tag game is about being on the ball, thinking fast and having fun.

AGE: 6–11 years (Year 2–Year 6)
POSTURES: Frog
SKILLS: Thinking, tactics, concentration, listening, communicating
RESOURCES: Cones for the line, game and posture cards

LEARNING OUTCOMES

> Can I improve *Frog Posture*?
> Can I travel in *Frog Posture*?
> Can I follow the rules of the game?

What to do

Choose someone to be the 'fleeing frog'.

The rest of the class squats in *Frog Posture*, in a straight line, down the centre of the hall. Alternate 'frogs' face in opposite directions as in the diagram. Make sure there is space at each end of the line so that the fleeing frog can get through.

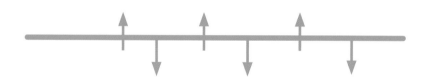

Choose someone to be the 'frog catcher'.

The frog catcher tries to catch fleeing frog. Frog catcher can only hop along one side of the line, whereas fleeing frog is allowed to hop on either side of the line, *but is not allowed to cross the line*. In other words he can only hop around it.

When fleeing frog hops around the line, frog catcher cannot follow. Instead she can tap the shoulder of one of the frogs that is facing the side to which fleeing frog has gone. That frog then becomes the new catcher and the old catcher takes his place in line. If fleeing frog is caught, choose a new fleeing frog and frog chaser. Does that make sense?

Repeat two to three times – no more because it's a killer!

FRONT TO FRONT

This is a great game for getting children to work with a variety of classmates – not just the usual suspects. Also you can squeeze lots of postures into this game. But the main point of the game is to encourage children to help each other in the posture.

AGE: 6–11 years (Year 2–Year 6)
POSTURES: Stick, Flamingo, Tree, Banana, Dancer 1, Dragon
SKILLS: Balancing, working with a partner, concentration, listening, communicating
RESOURCES: Game card and posture cards

LEARNING OUTCOMES

› Can I improve my partner work?
› Can I improve balance postures?
› Can I help my partner improve their balance?

What to do

Children walk around hall. You call out 'front to front' and the posture you want the children to take, for example, *Flamingo*.

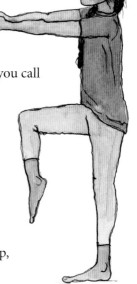

The children get into pairs, facing each other in the posture. Look out for opportunities to praise 'mirroring'.

Call all 'out change' and the children walk around again till you call out 'front to front' and the next posture, for example, *Tree*. At which point the children quickly find a *new* partner and stand facing each other in *Tree*. Again, look out for opportunities to praise 'mirroring'.

As children become more confident give fresh instructions including: back to back, elbow to elbow, side to side, toe to toe, finger to finger, knee to knee, hand to hand, and shoulder to shoulder, and so on.

Mix them up too, for example, finger to shoulder, knee to hip, front to back, etc.

Encourage children to help their partner and at the end of the lesson ask the children to nominate those who have been helpful. Perhaps ask them to show how they helped and were helped.

HEROES

This game is perfect for encouraging children to think about tactics, use of space and cooperation. Plus the fact that *Hero 2* is a very demanding posture and tag games are great fun so this is a winner.

AGE: 8–11 years (Year 4–Year 6)
POSTURES: Hero 2
SKILLS: Thinking, teamwork, listening, communicating
RESOURCES: Game card and posture cards

LEARNING OUTCOMES
> Can I avoid being caught?
> Can I hold *Hero 2* posture?
> Can I find tactics that will help me?

What to do
Choose a small team of, say, five children to be heroes. Give them a moment to have a tactics meeting. They position themselves separately across the hall in *Hero Posture*. They are allowed to pivot around on one foot providing they keep in posture.

The rest of the class run or walk quickly across the hall trying to get as close to the heroes without getting tagged. The heroes, being able to pivot on one foot, try to tag anyone near. If a hero tags anyone, they are captured and join up with their hero holding their trailing hands or using a band or tie (it helps each hero to be more pivotal).

Soon we have chains of heroes across the hall. As the chain grows, more people will be caught.

Repeat with a new starting team of heroes.

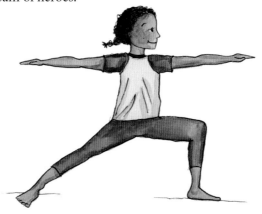

HERO IN THE CORNER

This game is noisy, energetic and contains the challenging *Hero* range of postures. No surprise that this game is so popular. Yet it is also a great opportunity to encourage the class to help each other in the posture.

AGE: 7–11 (Year 4–Year 6)
POSTURES: Hero 1, Hero 2, Hero 3 and Hero 4
SKILLS: Thinking, teamwork, listening, helping, communicating
RESOURCES: Large dice, four signs or cards labelled 1–4, game and posture cards

LEARNING OUTCOMES

> Can I be quietly focused in the *Hero Postures?*
> Can I help someone improve his or her posture?
> Can I guess the probability of the dice?

What to do

Demonstrate the four postures *Hero 1, 2, 3* and *4*. Put signs in each corner of the hall showing the numbers one, two, three and four. Ask the class to walk around the hall in a clockwise direction. When you call out 'hero' each person decides which corner to go to.

If, for example, someone goes to corner 1, then they are to come into *Hero 1 Posture*. Corner 2, into *Hero 2 Posture*, and so on.

Once they are quietly in posture you roll the dice. If the dice comes up two, then all people in corner 2 (i.e. *Hero 2*) are out of the game and come and sit in the middle of the circle of mats. Thus the game proceeds.

If you roll a five or six, then anyone who was out of the game is back in. The object of the game is to get out as many as possible…but it never happens because of the odds of fives and sixes coming up, which is why it is a great game to play with Years 5 and 6 to demonstrate probability.

The hero postures are challenging, so spend a little time beforehand finding ways that the children can help others with the postures. For example, holding the extended arms of a classmate in *Hero 1*. You do not need to be a yoga expert for this because it is just common sense.

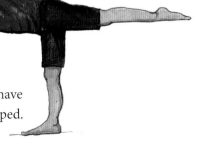

In the plenary, invite people to compliment those who have helped them in the posture, perhaps showing how they helped. You cannot beat practical demonstration!

HOOP GAME

Children adore this game. It's fast moving, addictive and I love it because we get to practise four postures in a short space of time. Furthermore you can play this game with children from Year 1 to Year 6, which is brilliant! With the older children capitalise on opportunities to demonstrate how to ask assertively to share space in the hoop. Trust me, opportunities will come up.

AGE: 5–11 years (Year 1–Year 6)
POSTURES: Frog, Chips, Flamingo, Dog, Hero, Crab…the choice is yours…just choose four
SKILLS: Thinking, teamwork, listening, helping, communicating
RESOURCES: Hoops – four each of green, yellow, blue and red. Game and posture cards

LEARNING OUTCOMES
> Can I perform the postures quietly focused?
> Can I follow the rules of the game?

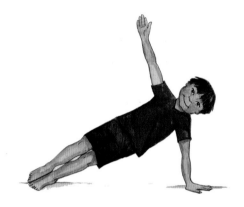

What to do
If you are playing with the whole class in the hall you will need four hoops of each colour; namely, red, blue, green and yellow. Have a corner for each colour spreading them out touching in the Olympic pattern.

Introduce (teach) or reinforce the postures if they already know them.

Have the children walking around the hall. When you yell 'HOOP!' each child chooses which colour, and therefore posture, to be in.

Another adult (or sensible child) who has their back to the action will, upon your signal, choose one of the four colours and give arbitrary points between one and five. Children in hoops of that colour will be very happy to hear that they have got points.

Carry on for another three or four rounds.

Alternative
Play a knock out game, that is, children in or around the yellow hoop are out of the game if yellow is called and will need to sit in *Good Sitting* on a mat. This should be fast and furious.

JIGSAW GAME

This game has 'the lot'. You can introduce new postures or reinforce 'old' ones. Plus the children practise teamwork skills such as listening, making sure everyone is included, resolving disputes as well as their presentation skills. You can expect some stunning group postures.

AGE: 7–11 years (Year 3–Year 6)
POSTURES: Stick, Chips, Tree, Boat, Flamingo, Banana, Frog, Hero, Candle, Tiger, Dancer 1
SKILLS: Teamwork, listening, helping, communicating
RESOURCES: Yoga at school jigsaws – see Resources page 91, game card

LEARNING OUTCOMES

> Can I cooperate with other children in my group?
> Can I listen to other children on my group?

What to do

Arrange the class into five groups of maximum six children. Each group selects a jigsaw bag from the box. Explain that, on your command, each group will work as a team to assemble the nine-piece jigsaw. When the jigsaw is complete they will need to use their team skills and their creative skills to create an interesting group posture.

Explain that they are expected to use their cooperation skills during the assembly of the jigsaw *and* the creation of the group posture.

Talk about those skills beforehand so they know what is expected.

Start them off and visit each group to offer encouragement.

Have each group perform their group posture to the class and ask them how they got on using their group skills.

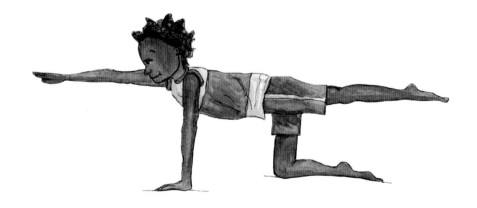

MAKE 'EM LAUGH

This is a simple game that is such fun and highly demanding on children because they have to try not to laugh, and also because in *Frog Posture* there is a lot going on in terms of strengthening and toning knees, ankles, toes and legs generally.

AGE: 6–11 years (Year 2–Year 6)
POSTURES: Frog
SKILLS: Listening, self-control
RESOURCES: Cones, game and posture cards

LEARNING OUTCOMES
> Can I keep going in *Frog Posture*?
> Can I control my urge to laugh?

What to do

Mark out a circuit with cones. Ask the children to come into *Frog Posture*.

Explain that they are to hop in *Frog Posture* around the circuit until you shout out 'STOP!'

They are to stop and be still and silent as 'frog statues'.

Your job is then to choose your 'victim' and try to make them laugh. Their job is not to laugh by controlling themselves. This applies to the whole class. If anyone laughs you get one point. If no one laughs they get the point.

Two circuits around the hall is fantastic exercise; three is a killer.

Add up the points, see who is the winner.

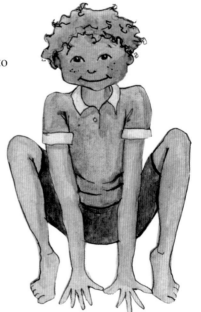

MIXING GAME

A brilliant team game where children combine two postures into one and discover a rich vein of creativity in their yoga and language work.

AGE: 6–11 years (Year 2–Year 6)
POSTURES: As many as possible
SKILLS: Listening, self-control, teamwork, language skills
RESOURCES: Game card and plenty of posture cards

LEARNING OUTCOMES

> Can I improve my teamwork skills?
> Can I create a new posture from two postures that I know?
> Can I think of a name for the new posture?

What to do

Split them into groups of five or six children. Each group chooses unseen two posture cards at random. At the given signal each group has a few minutes to combine the two postures into one, and invent an interesting name for the new posture. Remind the children that you are looking to reward teamwork skills, for example, listening and working together. Each group, in turn, performs their new posture and the rest of class has to guess the original two postures.

Here are some Year 5/6 examples:

◆ *Dragon + Boat = Dragboat*
◆ *Tree + Banana = Treeana*
◆ *Cobra +Chips = Chipcob*
◆ *Frog + Banana = Froganana*
◆ *Frog + Boat = Froat*
◆ *Banana + Dog = Banog*

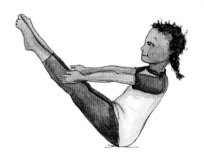
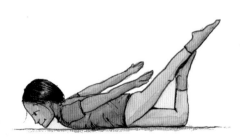

POISON

The fun in this game comes with the teasing use of words beginning with the letter 'P'. For example, 'I was…proudly walking in the…park on Sunday when a…pigeon landed on some…purple flowers. 'Stop,' I shouted, 'they may contain…poison!'

AGE: 6–11 years (Year 2–Year 6)
POSTURES: Tree, Flamingo
SKILLS: Balancing, storytelling, reacting quickly, listening
RESOURCES: Game and posture cards

LEARNING OUTCOMES

> Can I stand in *Tree* for a few minutes?
> Can I improvise a simple story?

What to do

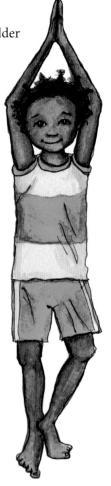

Have the whole class standing in *Tree Posture* in a tight circle, shoulder to shoulder with the yoga mats in an outer circle beyond.

You place yourself in the middle of the circle because you are the first storyteller. This enables you to model what you want the children to do.

You begin your story about anything often using words that begin with 'p'. At some point you will include the word 'poison'. At that point the children rush to a mat in the outer circle for safety.

The first person tagged by you before they can reach the safety of a mat is the next storyteller.

Repeat four or five times.

Extensions

Alternate postures. For example, *Tree, Flamingo, Tree*. Include any postures you consider suitable. Make sure the children are in postures that enable them to see and hear what is going on and can hold them easily for a while.

POSTURE IN THE BAG

This game is BAGS OF FUN. Pun intended. I often use the bags on fund-raising days when children have to guess which member of staff is in posture in the bag.

AGE: 6–11 years (Year 2–Year 6)
POSTURES: Variety
SKILLS: Questioning, performing, observing
RESOURCES: Large Lycra bags, game and posture cards

LEARNING OUTCOMES

> Can I use observation skills?
> Can I use my detective skills?

What to do

OPTION 1

Choose a child to secretly choose a posture.

Ask that child to get inside the bag and perform the posture. The rest of the class have three chances to guess the posture and perform it.

OPTION 2

As above in groups of five or six children.

OPTION 3

On special fund-raising days recruit other staff or children from other classes to appear in the bag. They can then lead the *Sun Sequence*. Children can have three guesses who is in the bag. You may need to provide some clues. For example, colour of hair, boy/girl, famous in school for singing, football, acting, etc.

PRISONERS

Children *are* competitive. So here is a game where you can harness that competiveness, practise *Eagle* and *Flamingo* postures and have lots of fun.

AGE: 8–11 years (Year 4–Year 6)
POSTURES: Eagle, Flamingo
SKILLS: Listening, concentrating, reacting quickly
RESOURCES: Game card and posture cards

LEARNING OUTCOMES
> Can I keep my concentration in *Eagle* and *Flamingo* postures?
> Can I devise a good tactic?

What to do
Split the class into two teams. Call them Team A and Team B. Have the two teams facing each other from opposite ends of the hall.

Have Team B go into *Flamingo* and Team A into *Eagle*.

Select a person from Team A to go to Team B and touch the fingertips of three members of Team B. As soon as he touches the fingertips of that third person, call her 'the thirdee'. He must run back to his own team without being caught by the thirdee.

If he is caught he becomes Team B's prisoner and has to stand behind Team B's line.

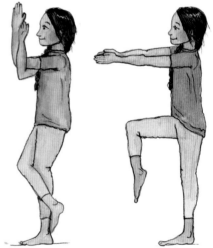

If he does not get caught, the thirdee becomes Team A's prisoner. Team B then goes into Eagle and Team A into Flamingo position and repeat the process.

Prisoners are released every time their team is successful.

At the end of the game the winner is the team with the most prisoners.

Extension
Play with *Hero 2* and *Hero 3 Postures*.

QUEENIE, QUEENIE

Hero 3 is a strong posture that helps to build strength in muscles. The 'Queenie, Queenie' song lasts long enough for children to hold the posture.

AGE: 8–11 years (Year 4–Year 6)
POSTURES: Hero 3
SKILLS: Concentrating, participating and listening
RESOURCES: Small ball, game card and posture card

LEARNING OUTCOMES
› Can I hold my concentration in *Hero 3*?
› Can I participate successfully?

What to do
Teach the class *Hero 3 Posture*.

The children form a circle and come into *Hero 3 Posture*. The teacher stands in the centre of the circle, with his eyes closed, holding a small ball, which he throws blindly over his shoulder.

The nearest child to where the ball lands, retrieves the ball and hides it in cupped hands *in Hero 3 Posture*.

All the class sing together:
> *Queenie, queenie who's got the ball?*
> *Are they thin or are they tall?*
> *Queenie, queenie who's got the ball?*

The teacher has three guesses to find who's got the ball.

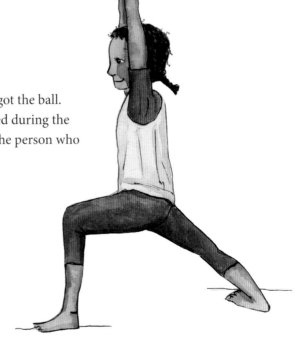

Encourage the class to be still and focused during the game, and to keep that leading knee bent. The person who has the ball can be the 'guesser' next time.

Repeat three times.

Extension
Use two balls – it's a bit crazy, but great fun.

ROCK PAPER SCISSORS

This all-time favourite is perfect for teaching cooperation and team skills, and can develop into a clever non-verbal game. I have yet to find a class who do not know how to play *Rock Paper Scissors*, so you will not need much input.

AGE: 8–11 years (Year 4–Year 6)
POSTURES: Flamingo, Tiger and Dragonfly
SKILLS: Concentrating, listening, group decision-making, working together, communicating verbally and non-verbally
RESOURCES: Game card and posture cards

LEARNING OUTCOMES
> Can I improve my teamwork skills?
> Can I perform *Dragonfly, Tiger* and *Flamingo Postures* as part of a group?

What to do
Show children the three posture cards that are involved in the game and how it works. For example, *Tiger* beats *Flamingo*, *Flamingo* beats *Dragonfly*, *Dragonfly* beats *Tiger*.

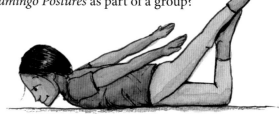

It will help the children to understand if you set the cards in a triangle shape, and have them where they can be seen as a reminder. Divide the whole class into two teams, each with an adult in charge. Each team huddles down to choose *one* posture. Look for opportunities to highlight good listening, children cooperating, and encourage and praise children staying calm even when they disagree with others. Try voting for the posture and using appropriate vocabulary like *majority*, *being fair*, and so on.

Each team then forms a straight line facing each other (mats could mark out where you want to the teams to be). Choose someone to say 'ready steady go' and everyone gets into posture at the same time. Winners gain one point. Encourage the losers to congratulate the winners. Call everyone back into their team huddles and repeat at least three rounds.

Extensions
- Stage 1: No adult team leaders – leave the children to sort themselves out.
- Stage 2: No verbal communication allowed, but do allow posture cards.
- Stage 3: No verbal communication allowed and no use of posture cards.

SHARK GAME

Shark Game is a great favourite for the children, and a highly versatile game for you. It's a game of contrasts: screaming to silence; fast movement to stillness and focus.

AGE: 5–11 years (Year 1–Year 6)
POSTURES: Tree, Flamingo and Dragon
SKILLS: Balancing, focusing, self-control
RESOURCES: Game card and posture cards

LEARNING OUTCOMES

> Can I make *Tree Feet*?
> Can I stretch up in *Tree/Dragon Posture*?
> Can I focus on an object in *Tree/Dragon/Flamingo Posture*?

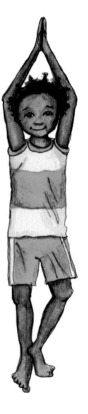

What to do

Set up mats in a circle in the hall. Have the whole class standing in *Stick Posture* on their mats.

Ask them to come into the water (i.e. the floor) and pretend to be swimming. Encourage children to use their shoulders and their arms fully. To avoid bumping, have everyone 'swimming' in the same direction.

When you shout 'SHARK!' each child will have to get to a mat for safety and stand in *Tree Posture*, calmly focused. Anyone not on a mat, or with a 'toe in the water', or talking has to go and lie down on the shark's dinner table. This can be an area in the centre of the circle or wherever you decide.

Repeat four or five times.

Extensions

◆ You could alternate postures, for example, *Tree*, *Dragon* and *Tree*. Include any postures you consider suitable. Make sure the children are in postures that enable them to see and hear what is going on.

◆ If you are using coloured mats, you could make a rule that no one is allowed on a blue mat, then purple, and so on. Eventually you will have the class trying to stand calmly on three mats. This is excellent for encouraging children to share a small space. Or you could put bean bags on mats that are 'out of bounds'.

◆ Try tricking children into speaking by asking questions.

SNEAKY TREES

All children adore this classic game based on 'Grandma's Footsteps'. This is the game that will reinforce *Tree Posture*, will help children get to grips with balancing and encourage them to learn how to be still and focused. Without doubt this game is the most popular and most effective yoga game in the world.

AGE: 4–11 years (Nursery–Year 6)
POSTURES: Tree
SKILLS: Balancing, focusing, self-control
RESOURCES: Game card and posture card

LEARNING OUTCOMES

> Can I stand in *Tree Feet*?
> Can I stretch my branches (arms up)?
> Can I stand very still and quietly focused in *Tree Posture*?
> Can I follow instructions?

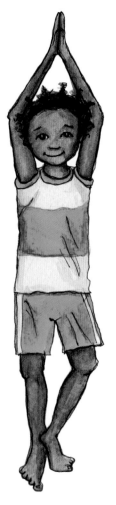

What to do

Children stand in *Stick Position* on their mats facing into the centre of the circle. Position yourself at the centre of the circle. Show the children how you want them to slowly tiptoe towards you at the centre, emphasising the slow tiptoe movements. On the 'go' signal, the children tiptoe slowly forward. The teacher calls out 'sneaky trees' and children come into *Tree Posture* quietly, calmly and focused. Look out for opportunities to compliment children on the three important aspects of the *Tree Posture*, that is, *Tree Feet*, hands stretching up and their calm focus on a specific object.

Repeat three times.

Extensions

◆ Straight line: Have the children stand in a straight line on one side of the hall (use a long rope as a guide). Repeat as above.

◆ What are you focused on?: Position various interesting objects in their eyeline that the children can focus on. Encourage them to focus on one of the objects when they are in *Tree Posture*. It makes it more fun if the teacher has to guess which object a child is focused on.

◆ Nail, tightrope and mud game: This is a big favourite. Repeat as above. Pretend that you have scattered sharp nails in the way and the children have to act out what happens when they step on the sharp nails. Of course, when you shout 'sneaky trees', they have to stop and stand quietly focused in *Tree Posture*. Repeat with 'tightrope' and 'mud'. It is a game of great contrasts…the excitement of walking through mud, over nails and along the tightrope compared to the stillness and concentration in *Tree Posture*.

STICK BALL GAME

Surprisingly simple and popular, this game is very good for encouraging children to stand quietly still.

AGE: 6–11 years (Year 2–Year 6)
POSTURES: Stick
SKILLS: Self-control, standing quietly
RESOURCES: Game card and posture card

LEARNING OUTCOMES

⟩ Can I stand very still and quietly focused in *Stick Posture*?
⟩ Can I follow the rules of the game?

What to do

This game is faster and better with small groups, so split the class into groups of five or six children.

Everyone stands in *Stick Posture* in a small circle. Adjust the posture so that arms and hands are behind backs.

One child is chosen to stand in the middle of the small circle either blindfolded or on a promise to keep his eyes closed.

Children pass a small ball around the circle. At some point one of the children in the circle hides the ball behind her back. The person in the middle opens his eyes and has two or three guesses who has the ball.

Everyone needs to be standing quietly in *Stick Posture*.

Choose another to go in the centre and continue the game.

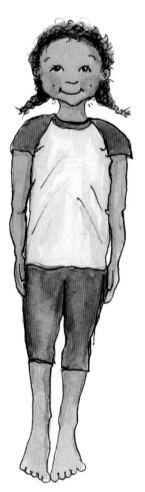

SPIN THE POSTURE

Children love games that involve an element of silent, drawn-out suspense as they wait to discover whether they will be victor or victim. This game can involve as many postures as you like, and demonstrates to children that they have the skills to control their bodies, minds and voice when necessary.

AGE: 6–11 years (Year 2–Year 6)
POSTURES: Hero 3, Flamingo, Boat, Tiger, Dancer and Dragon – whatever you choose
SKILLS: Self-control, concentration, listening, and following the rules of the game
RESOURCES: Spinning wheel, game and posture cards

LEARNING OUTCOMES
> Can I quietly concentrate in each posture?
> Can I work out the probability of what comes next?
> Can I follow the rules of the game?

What to do
Set out seven posture cards in the order one to seven where they can be seen.

You shout out 'NOW!' Each child decides which posture to come into from those shown, doing their best to remain silent, still and focused.

There is now a short period of absolute silence during which you spin the wheel of your spinner. When the number comes up you announce it, at the same time awarding points, depending on the difficulty of the posture.

Repeat for another three or four rounds. See who has the most points. Though point out that it doesn't matter 'We are just having fun practising our postures'.

Valuable Teaching Tip 1: You could make or buy a large spinner that shows all the postures and where the arrow lands.
Valuable Teaching Tip 2: No spinner? How about a large dice and call the game: *Roll the Posture.*

TWO TREES TAG

Pair work is good for cooperation skills and learning how to get on better. Tag games are great fun. So, by combining the two, children get the best of both worlds as well as practising an important balance posture.

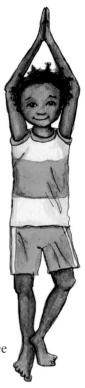

AGE: 7–11 years (Year 3–Year 6)
POSTURES: Tree, Boat and Flamingo
SKILLS: Cooperation, tactics and communicating
RESOURCES: Game card and posture cards

LEARNING OUTCOMES
› Can I cooperate well in twos and threes?
› Can I follow the rules of the game?

What to do
Children get into pairs on a mat and link up in *Tree Posture*.

Choose two children to run around: one chasing, the other fleeing. If the fleer gets caught he becomes the chaser and chases the now new fleer.

The fleer can join up with one of the pairs in *Tree Posture*, which means that the person furthest away from the new arrival in *Tree* now becomes the new fleer and has to run around looking to join another tree pair and dislodge one of the pair. It's fast and furious and great fun.

Extensions
Try different postures that lend themselves well to pair work. For example, *Boat*, *Flamingo* or *Banana*.

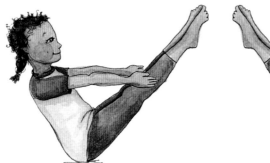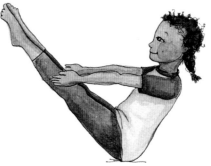

THREE STEP STICK

This game is about giving children the opportunity and reason to stand still for a short time. This game is harder than it sounds.

AGE: 8–11 years (Year 4–Year 6)
POSTURES: Stick, Frog
SKILLS: Cooperation, thinking, tactics, listening
RESOURCES: Game card and posture cards

LEARNING OUTCOMES

> Can I follow the rules of the game with honesty?
> Can I stand quietly in *Stick Posture*?

What to do

Chose one child to be 'it'. That child is blindfolded. The rest of the class spreads out across the hall and stands very still in *Stick Posture*.

The blindfolded child roams the hall with his arms flailing trying to tag someone.

The children are allowed *three* steps to escape from being caught. They can use their three steps in the following ways: either one or two at a time or all in one go.

Either way, once they have used their three steps, that's it, they cannot move again.

They can also squat down into *Frog Posture* to avoid being tagged.

When someone is tagged they become 'it' and the game starts over.

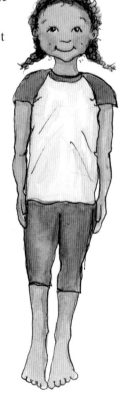

Helpful Hint: Have someone guiding the blindfolded child.

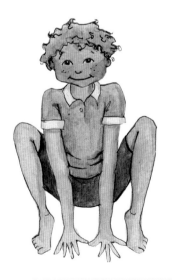

TOILET GAME

This is a tag team game which is great fun. All my classes love this game and beg to play it every week so I keep it up my sleeve for a special treat. The slow motion element adds to the fun and helps children be more aware of their body movement.

AGE: 8–11 years (Year 4–Year 6)
POSTURES: Toilet, Flushing toilet
SKILLS: Cooperation, thinking, tactics, listening
RESOURCES: Game card and posture cards

LEARNING OUTCOMES

> Can I demonstrate the *Toilet* and *Flushing Toilet Postures*?
> Can I think up tactics that help me avoid being caught?

What to do

Your first task is to teach the children the two postures, which are: *Toilet Posture* and *Flushing Toilet Posture*.

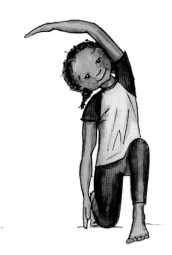

Choose three children to be the taggers; the rest of the class walk around the hall in slow motion. The taggers meanwhile can *walk* around at *normal walking pace*.

When a child is tagged she comes into *Toilet Posture*.

Another child can release her by flushing her…and off she goes, back in the game.

It is a fast physical game so I tend to shout out 'freeze!' after 40 seconds and change the taggers so that everyone gets to be in posture.

Repeat three or four times and move on to the next stage of the lesson – leave them wanting more.

WHAT'S THE TIME MR WOLF?

This is a game of great contrasts. Contrasts between the excitement and screaming and running around trying not to be caught, and the stillness and silence of standing in *Stick Posture*. Children get to practise four or five postures too.

AGE: 3–7 years (Nursery–Year 2)
POSTURES: (For example) Stick, Tree, Flamingo, Chips and Frog. You choose, but Stick is obligatory
SKILLS: Concentration, listening, following instructions
RESOURCES: Game card and posture cards

LEARNING OUTCOMES

› Can I be still and quiet in *Stick* after being noisy?
› Am I alert?
› Can I follow instructions?

What to do

Ask the class to walk about in the hall. They are to ask you: 'What's the time Mr Wolf?'

You reply, for example: 'It's Tree time', meaning that everyone comes into *Tree Posture*. Holding up the posture card helps too.

Repeat this a couple of times with other postures, for example, *Flamingo* and *Chips*. Finally, you answer 'Dinner time!' whereupon everyone has to get to the mat to be safe from the wolf. Once on the mat children need to stand still and quietly in *Stick Posture*.

Repeat two or three times.

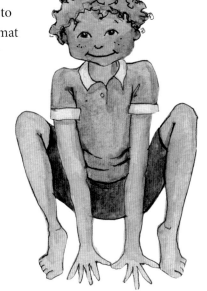

Extension

Choose a sensible child to be the wolf.

YOGA RELAY GAME

This typical relay game is fast, furious and great fun. Travelling in *Dog*, *Crab* and *Tree* is terrific exercise and an interesting contrast to postures that are normally static.

AGE: 8–11 years (Year 4–Year 6)
POSTURES: Dog, Crab and Tree work well as travelling postures – you choose
SKILLS: Teamwork, travelling in the postures and following instructions
RESOURCES: Game card and posture cards

LEARNING OUTCOMES

> Can I move quickly in *Dog*, *Crab* and *Tree*?
> Am I alert?
> Can I follow instructions?

What to do

Set out two marker cones opposite each other and a good distance between them for *each* team, i.e. six cones. Use three colours, for example, blue, red and yellow.

A   B

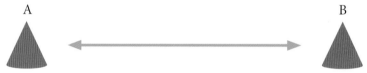

Divide the class into three teams: blue, red and yellow. Ideally there should be around ten in each team, or whatever number suits your class.

Half of each team lines up behind one of their respective coloured cones and the other half behind their opposite cone.

Decide the running order of the postures, for example, *Dog*, *Crab*, *Tree*, and be clear which children will be starting first, those at A or B.

On the word 'GO!' the starters at A travel in *Dog Posture* to the opposite cone, B. As soon as they reach it, their opposite number comes back in *Crab*. As soon as *Crab* reaches cone A, *Tree* hops to B. And so it continues. When someone completes their turn they sit in *Good Sitting* at the back of their line.

The winners are the first team finished quietly in *Good Sitting* with their hands in the air.

Repeat twice more.

Extension

Change the order of the postures.

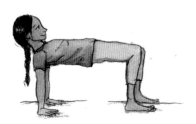

YOGLIE, BOGLIE, MOGLIE

Here is a simple game that is noisy, fast moving, frantic and great fun. Yet in the middle of the madness children are standing in posture quietly focused. Amazing!

AGE: 8–11 years (Year 4–Year 6)
POSTURES: Stick, Tree, Chips, Hero 2 and Dragon work well – you choose or mix it up a bit
SKILLS: Following instructions, concentration
RESOURCES: Game card and posture cards

LEARNING OUTCOMES

> Can I be still and quiet in *Stick* after being noisy?
> Am I alert?
> Can I follow instructions?

What to do

Children stand in *Chips* or *Tree Posture*, or any standing posture that they can sustain for a longish time.

Approach a child and say: 'Yoglie, Boglie, Moglie', whereupon that child must leave his mat and he in turn can displace another child from her mat by saying: 'Yoglie, Boglie, Moglie'. And so it goes on.

At any point you call out 'stop-freeze!' Anyone not on a mat is out of the game.

It's even more exciting when you have several displaced children running around trying to get on to a mat.

Run the game for around 5 minutes. They will appreciate calming and relaxation after this.

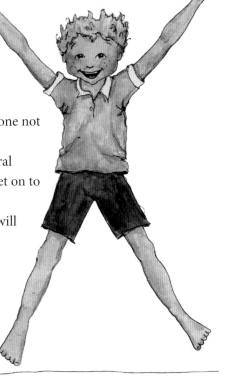

CALMING GAMES

RAINSTICK GAME

This is one of the most successful games to help children become still and calm. It works well because most children want to be chosen and the rainstick sound in the silence of the class is calming and magical.

AGE: 4–11 years (Reception–Year 6)
POSTURES: Good Sitting
SKILLS: Sitting quietly focused
RESOURCES: Good quality long rainstick, game card

LEARNING OUTCOMES
› Can I sit in *Good Sitting* with a straight back?
› Can I keep my eyes closed and listen?

What to do
Children sit quietly on chairs (or mats) in *Good Sitting*.
Choose someone as a good example who has all the attributes you are looking for:

◆ straight backs
◆ thumb and index finger touching
◆ warm friendly smile (optional)
◆ most importantly, his eyes are gently closed.

Tiptoe up to your good example and invert the rainstick near his ear so that he can clearly hear the trickling rain sound.

Explain that he will now choose someone to take the rainstick to…that he will only choose someone with a straight back, eyes closed.

Repeat four times asking children to be fair and not to choose their friends.

Keep stressing that anyone peeping will not be chosen.

RELAXATION

LADYBIRD RELAXATION

Your pupils will look forward to this, will complain if, for any reason, you leave it out, and they will forever tell you how they use this relaxation outside of the yoga lesson. Which is good news, because relaxation calms busy minds and the young nervous systems, which in turn helps children deal with anxiety and tension and ultimately reduces stress.

AGE: 4–11 years (Reception–Year 6)
POSTURES: Supine (lying on your back)
SKILLS: Being quietly calm yet focused
RESOURCES: Ladybird puppet, bells, game card

LEARNING OUTCOMES

> Can I lay still in *Ladybird Relaxation Posture* on my mat?
> Can I keep my eyes closed?
> Can I imagine the ladybird landing on my different body parts?

What to do

Have the children lie on mats on their backs – which is a supine position – with their arms by their sides, palms upwards. Or be in *Good Sitting* in their chairs.

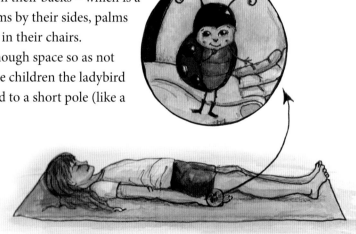

Make sure each child has enough space so as not to disturb anyone else. Show the children the ladybird finger puppet on string attached to a short pole (like a fishing rod).

Let the children know that the ladybird will only land on children who are lying very still.

Ask the children to close

their eyes gently and to imagine that the tiny, shy ladybird is flying around the hall/room and gently landing on… (the 'script' is below – feel free to change it to suit your class' needs).

The key

The key to this is to use a strong, yet warm, calm voice. Often, when I introduce this technique for the first 3–4 weeks I ask the children to think about how the tiny, shy ladybird may be feeling, that any movement may frighten or startle the ladybird and to show me how kind they can be by being as still as they can. It's a motivation that works well. Try it!

Structure and route

Other key aspects to this technique are that the ladybird takes *the same route each time.* It can be clockwise or anti-clockwise. Rarely do I use the words left or right because that can be confusing for many children. I prefer to use the words 'the *other* shoulder, thumb, toe' instead. By keeping to the structure each time you will reinforce the activity, which helps your children learn to a degree that they can practise this on their own at home or, frankly, anywhere.

Bells

I also suggest that you use a simple triangle that you ding each time the ladybird lands on a body part. The gentle sound seems to help the children focus; continuously striking the triangle signals the end of the relaxation.

Expectations

Do set your expectations at realistic levels: there will be some children who will fidget to some degree. That's normal. You will find, though, that they are fidgeting a lot less than they normally would, and through regular practice fidgeting and most movement will disappear – so persevere!

Ladybird relaxation script

A tiny, shy, tired ladybird needs to find somewhere safe to rest for a while. She/he looks down and sees you lying so still and calm. She/he thinks you look kind so she/he lands carefully on…
Your big toe, and stays for a moment.
Then ladybird flaps its wings and flies in the air and lands gently…
On your knee, and stays for another moment.
Ladybird flaps its wings again, flies in the air and lands softly…

On the tip of your thumb, and stays for a moment there too.

Ladybird flaps its wings again, flies in the air and lands softly on…

Your shoulder, happy to stay there for a moment.

Ladybird flaps its wings and flies in the air and this time lands gently on…

The tip of your nose, and stays for a tiny moment sharing your stillness.

Ladybird flaps its wings and flies in the air and lands softly on…

Your other shoulder, and is so comfortable that she/he stays for another moment.

Ladybird flaps its wings and flies in the air and lands carefully on…

Your other thumb, she/he is so happy to share your calmness she/he stays for a few moments more.

Ladybird flaps its wings and flies in the air and lands softly on…

Your other knee, where she stays just for another moment, very still, like you.

Ladybird flaps its wings and flies in the air and lands carefully on…

Your other big toe, and settles down quietly, calmly and happily.

Allow the children to relax *in silence* for up to 1–2 minutes. Trust your judgement to bring them up when you think the time is right. Complete the relaxation by saying:

And then the ladybird flaps its wings and flies away, back to its home in the trees.

Allow and enjoy a few more moments of silence as the children re-orientate themselves.

NURSERY GAMES

I love teaching yoga to nursery classes because the children are honest and funny and crazy.

However, I would not love it if I made the cardinal mistake of using a story approach with them. The key to successful yoga lessons with nursery classes is always…

Structure

Structure

Structure.

A story approach does not lend itself easily to structure. You would need to be a highly experienced, ultraconfident nursery/drama teacher to use story and maintain control of the class. For sure, at the beginning of term when everything is new and daunting to many of the children, structure, continuity and patience are essential to put them at their ease.

Having taught countless nursery classes, there is no doubt that the combination of tight structure, visual timetable, engaging fun games, clear achievable learning objectives and sufficient support from staff are what is required to teach yoga to nursery classes successfully. Never more so since classes contain an increasing diversity of nationalities, abilities and emerging special needs.

SET-UP

There are several factors that will determine how you set up the class.

The first factor is *class numbers*. If you teach a relatively small class, say 6–12 children, I suggest that you set up a circle of chairs in your classroom, for the following reasons:

- ◆ pupils are less inclined to run around, because the workspace is enclosed
- ◆ you will keep transition problems to the minimum
- ◆ pupils are familiar with chairs, and less inclined to fidget
- ◆ it is a 'base' to return to when a child has completed the posture
- ◆ it is easier to manage children waiting for their turn if they are seated.

Above all, this set-up will help children with emerging special needs.

Alternatively, children could be sitting on the carpet in a circle. No yoga mats yet!

Experiment to find what works best for your class. My guess is that if you have a high number of children showing emerging special needs, chairs will be the better option.

If class numbers are 15+ then the school hall will be best. You will have set up your colourful yoga mats in a circle. Initially it is challenging having 15 or more children filing in, sorting out shoes, socks and tights, and then finding a mat to sit on. Persevere, and by session three or four, most of them will know what to do. In any case it is good discipline for them.

STAFF RATIOS

The more adult staff members in the lesson the better.

One of my students, who was teaching yoga in a private nursery, asked me to observe her lesson because she was having class management problems. My student had been there for four weeks. Right from her first lesson staff at the nursery had been impressed with her professionalism. Unfortunately their attitude was: 'she knows what she's doing, kids are enjoying themselves we can have a tea break'.

So my poor student was left to cope with 15 nursery children single handedly. It was simple to suggest a remedy to improve class management. Staff participate. Help in the lesson. Have a tea break later.

ROLE OF STAFF IN THE LESSON

The key to the success and positive impact of the yoga lies squarely in the hands of the teaching staff. Their main responsibility is to ensure that the weekly 30-minute yoga lesson happens and that the lesson is delivered with enthusiasm, that everyone is challenged and achieves, and that there is a great sense of fun about the occasion.

More specifically staff will find themselves:

◆ modelling postures
◆ assisting children in postures
◆ taking some children through sequences
◆ singing the songs that accompany the postures and activities.

As well as encouraging pupils to:

◆ work independently
◆ anticipate movement

- wait their turn
- complete lines of song and join in songs.

STAGES OF THE LESSON

The stages I suggest for nursery are slightly different to the stages I suggest for Reception and upwards as shown on page 11. I suggest that you stick to the following structure for at least two terms.

Structure for first two terms (approx. 20 weeks):

1 beginning/development
2 sequence
3 relaxation
4 ending and exit.

You will note that the beginning and development stages have been merged. The reason is this: from the outset you will be training the children to start the lesson sitting quietly in *Good Sitting*. If the lesson is taking place in the classroom on chairs or the carpet, this will happen quickly. If you are filing into the hall it will take longer. Either way you cannot expect children of this age to sit still for long. Therefore, before they begin to fidget or talk, take action to engage them in the development activity.

By the third term you can revert to the stages that are as shown on page 11 because by that time the children will have developed the skills and understanding to deal with that structure and you will be preparing them for the structure they will face when they move up to Reception class.

BEGINNING GAMES/DEVELOPMENT

There are THREE main games to choose from, which are:

- Matching Game
- Umbrella Game
- Bean Bag Game.

The three games are similar in that they contain the same postures. Also every posture has a specific activity that makes the posture fun and engaging.

For example when you practise *Banana Posture* you will be singing along to the banana song. When you practise *Hero Posture* the children will be gripping the hero pole and singing along to the hero music, which is the theme to Indiana Jones, and therefore easy to remember.

In other words, each and every posture at this level has a specific activity. It is not just a matter of doing the posture. That would be dry and boring and the class would soon disengage. This is the key to successful lessons at this level.

The following chart shows you the activities that work best with the postures.

POSTURE	PRACTISED WITH...
Banana	The banana song I'm a banana, Oh I'm a banana, I'm a banana, nana, nana, nana, I'm a banana, oh I'm a banana, I'm a banana, nana, nana...noo
Hero	(Tune: Hum Theme from Indiana Jones. Da da dada dada) Use the Hero Pole to help children with balance.
Candle	Counting up to ten. Counting down from ten. Counting in French or Spanish.
Chips	The Chips Song: I love chips... I love Chips... I love chips... I love chips...and tomato ketchup.
Boat	(Tune: Row, Row, Row your Boat) Yo, yo yoga boat gently on the floor Merrily, Merrily, Merrily, Merrily we can do some more..
Tree	(Tune: Twinkle, Twinkle, Little Star) Tree Song: Tree feet, Tree arms , Tree eyes too. I can stand here all day through. Tree feet, Tree arms, Tree eyes too. (In a whisper)Balancing quietly, Hey, can you?
Frog	Hop up and down in Frog Posture saying Ribbet, Ribbet. When teacher stops, everyone stops and everyone is absolutely still like a frog statue. Anyone who does not is out of the game for a couple of turns. Repeat 3–4 times.
Dragon	(Tune: Frere Jacque) I'm in Dragon, I'm in Dragon, Look at me. Look at me, Stretching to the ceiling, Stretching to the ceiling, Well done me, Well done you.

MATCHING GAME

This game is ideal for introducing yoga to small nursery classes. Children will be practising simple, yet important skills and learning how to sit quietly for a short while.

AGE: 3–5 years (Nursery–Reception)
POSTURES: Hero, Banana, Boat, Candle, Frog, Chips, Dragon and Tree
SKILLS: Matching, taking turns/waiting, listening, participating, communicating
RESOURCES: Matching Game posture cards and matching board. See Resources page 91
NOTE: Add other postures when you feel children are ready.

LEARNING OUTCOMES

> Can I do the postures?
> Can I wait my turn?
> Can I sit in *Good Sitting*?
> Can I speak loudly?

What to do

Display Matching Game posture cards on a Velcro strip or portable visual timetable.

Select a pupil to come up to the display and select a card (help if necessary).

Hold up the matching board and give the pupil time to match it to the correct picture (again, help if necessary).

Ask her what it says, and ask her to shout out the name of the posture (model shouting the name of the posture).

Then the class should perform the posture.

Everyone goes back to their chairs.

Repeat until the game is complete.

Valuable Teaching Tip: If possible make it clear that those in *Good Sitting Posture* will be asked to choose from the display strip.

UMBRELLA GAME

What a game! This is one of the most successful Early Years/special needs yoga games – EVER! Playing will create loads of opportunities to encourage *Good Sitting*, taking turns, waiting patiently, joining in, completing sentences and decision-making

AGE: 3–5 years (Nursery–Reception)
POSTURES: Hero, Boat, Banana, Dragon, Candle, Frog, Chips and Tree
SKILLS: Matching, taking turns, waiting, listening, participating, communicating
RESOURCES: Umbrella, small posture cards, game card. See Resources, page 91
NOTE: As time goes by, add different postures

LEARNING OUTCOMES
› Can I wait my turn?
› Can I sit in *Good Sitting*?
› Can I speak loudly?
› Can I join in with the singing?

Make your umbrella...it's easy
First buy a safe children's umbrella from Mothercare/Toys "R" Us. Hang the posture cards inside the umbrella. Each posture is represented by a set of two identical cards velcroed back to back.

What to do
Encourage students to be in *Good Sitting* in the circle whether on chairs, the carpet or mats. Walk or skip around the inside of the circle singing the umbrella song twice:

> *Umbrella, umbrella please choose me*
> *I'm in Good Sitting*
> *Can you see?*

I tell the students that the umbrella is magic and that the magic ONLY works when everyone is quietly in *Good Sitting* with lovely straight backs (works a treat!).

   Choose someone who is trying his or her best in *Good Sitting* (that's the incentive!). Hold the umbrella above his head and let him choose from the selection of postures hanging down from inside of umbrella. He simply pulls off one card from the set.

I will encourage that child to shout out the name of the posture because, for many, it is an opportunity to punch through their shyness.

The whole class comes into the posture, OR children take turns demonstrating the posture – whatever you feel is most appropriate and works best within the constraints of your space.

Repeat with four or five postures, moving on before the children become restless.

BEAN BAG GAME

This game encourages throwing skills and fine motor skills as well as thinking skills and social skills like turn taking before you even get into the postures. For many students the chance to get to have a go at throwing the bean bag into a hole is a big incentive for engagement.

AGE: 3–5 years (Nursery–Reception)
POSTURES: Hero, Boat, Banana, Dragon, Candle, Frog, Chips and Tree
SKILLS: Taking turns/waiting, listening, participating, communicating
RESOURCES: Bean bag board, small bean bags, posture cards
NOTE: As time goes by add different postures

LEARNING OUTCOMES

> Can I wait my turn?
> Can I sit in *Good Sitting*?
> Can I speak loudly?
> Can I throw underarm?

What to do

Have an adult demonstrate how to throw a bean bag into one of the holes in the board and choose the posture. Then select a pupil to have a go. Some pupils may need help; some may need to drop the bean bag in the hole from no distance, or some may find the target from a distance. Having chosen the posture in this way practise the postures as in the Umbrella Game on page 86.

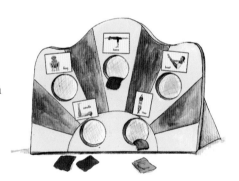

SEQUENCE

I call the sequence that I teach Nursery children *Sun Game*. This is more appropriate terminology at this level. *Sun Game* is easy to learn and fun, and serves as a foundation for more challenging sequences in later years.

When I introduce *Sun Game* to a new class I tend to teach them only the first four postures of the sequence in the first couple of sessions. That way it keeps things simple and easy to follow. When I deem they are ready I will teach them the rest of the *Sun Game*.

That said, there have been many times when I have taught the whole thing in Session 1. I encourage you to 'play it by ear'. Look back to page 31 for more details on how to play this.

RELAXATION

Relaxation for nursery children needs to be simple and as
unwordy as possible.

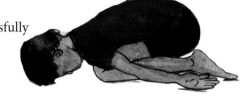

I have been using *Sleeping Bird* successfully
for years. I suggest that you keep it as the
relaxation part of your lesson for at least
two terms and then introduce *Ladybird
Relaxation* on page 79 in the third term.

When you are ready for this part of the lesson have the whole class curl down
in *Sleeping Bird* for 2–4 minutes. It will help if you sing – and keep singing – the
following song until the majority of children are in posture.

> *I'm curling down in Bird*
> *I'm curling down in Bird*
> *Hey ho everyone*
> *I'm curling down in Bird.*

Reduce to a whisper. Then to silence.

Throughout the time encourage the children to keep their eyes closed, and to be as
still as they can. I usually say: 'Show me how you can keep your head still…and your
arms…and your feet, and so on'. In other words, be directive – the children will find
that more than helpful. Try also to say the same thing every week. That reinforces the
activity, and helps nursery children feel secure.

Keep the children in *Bird* for as long as possible, but do not overstay your welcome.

Then, gently bring them out of posture by tapping their shoulder with a pole, for
example, saying '*Bird* is finished…sitting back in our chairs or lining up in *Stick* by
the door'.

RESOURCES

POSTURE AND GAME CARDS

The visual timetable together with Posture Cards and Game Cards are integral to my teaching approach and will, without doubt, improve the quality of your lessons and classroom management.

MAKE YOUR OWN OR BUY MINE?

You can make your own posture or game cards or you could save yourself a lot of time and energy by downloading mine at: www.yogaatschool.org.uk/game+posture+cards

As you have bought the book you can use the code chicken008 to claim your discount.

SONGS FOR NURSERY GAMES

You can access and listen to and download songs at the same page on the website. You will need to use the code chicken009 to obtain them for FREE at: www.yogaatschool.org.uk/game+posture+cards

The same goes for Matching Game. Make your own or download mine at: www. yogaatschool.org.uk/matching+game

Again, as you have bought the book you can use the code chicken010 to claim your discount.

YOGA JIGSAWS

Once again as a book buyer you are entitled to a discount on the range of wooden yoga jigsaws. Use the code chicken011 to claim it at the following link: www.yogaatschool. org.uk/yoga+jigsaws

OTHER RESOURCES

If you would like guidance on other resources for children's yoga feel free to contact me at: info@yogaatschool.org.uk

POSTURE CARDS AND GAMES CARDS TO START YOU OFF

To start you off here are the *Trees* Posture Card together with *Sneaky Trees* and *Shark* Game Cards, which you can cut out, laminate and use immediately.

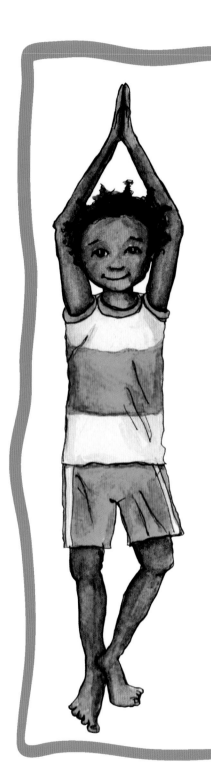

tree

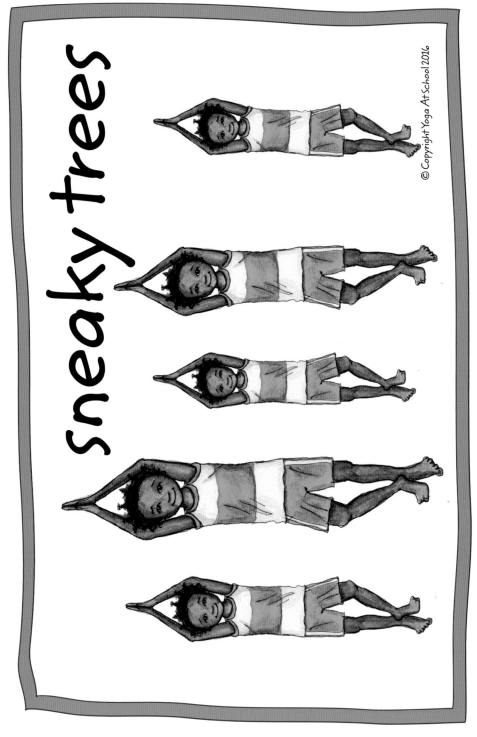

sneaky trees

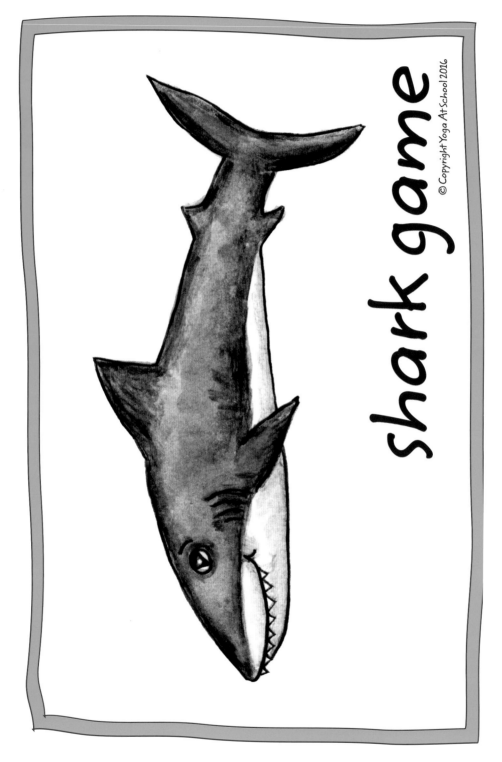

shark game

EASY WAYS TO CHOOSE GAMES

GAMES LIST

GAMES BY LESSON STAGE

BEGINNING GAMES

Banana Game
Beat the Clock
Good Sitting Game
Knock Down the Tower Game
Sitting on a Chicken
The Wrong Posture

SEQUENCE GAMES

Chase the Frog
One Behind
The Incredible Weather Game
Yoga Detective What's Missing?
Yoga Detective Who's Talking?
Yoga Detective Who's the Leader?

DEVELOPMENT GAMES

Brilliant Balancers
Butterfly Skittles
Chips in the Mud
Concentration/Matching Game –
in Small Groups
Concentration/Matching Game –
Whole Class
Crown Game
Dog Relay
Don't Be Sad
Flower Game

Fleeing Frog
Front to Front
Heroes
Hero in the Corner
Hoop Game
Jigsaw Game
Make 'Em Laugh
Mixing Game
Poison
Posture in the Bag
Prisoners
Queenie, Queenie
Rock Paper Scissors
Shark Game
Sneaky Trees
Stick Ball Game
Spin the Posture
Two Trees Tag
Three Step Stick
Toilet Game
What's the Time Mr Wolf?
Yoga Relay Game
Yoglie, Boglie, Moglie

CALMING GAMES

Rainstick Game

RELAXATION

Ladybird Relaxation

GAMES BY AGE

I have listed the games in line with the English educational system. For those of you in other countries you have a helpful guide to age range. Many games for younger children can be played with the older children. Simply adjust your language and increase the challenge. For example, *Shark Game*. In other words be adventurous and flexible, this is only a guide.

NURSERY-KINDERGARTEN (3-4 YEARS)

Bean Bag Game
Don't Be Sad
Good Sitting Game
Matching Game
Sneaky Trees
Umbrella Game
What's the Time Mr Wolf?

RECEPTION (4-5 YEARS)

Banana Game
Don't Be Sad
Good Sitting Game
Ladybird Relaxation
Rainstick Game
Sneaky Trees
What's the Time Mr Wolf?

YEAR 1 (5-6 YEARS)

Banana Game
Don't Be Sad
Good Sitting Game
Knock Down the Tower Game
Ladybird Relaxation
Rainstick Game
Shark Gameww
Sneaky Trees
What's the Time Mr Wolf?

YEAR 2 (6-7 YEARS)

Banana Game
Chase the Frog
Flower Game
Knock Down the Tower Game
Ladybird Relaxation
Rainstick Game
Shark Game
Sneaky Trees
Stick Ball Game
Yoga Detective What's Missing?

YEAR 3 (7-8 YEARS)

Banana Game
Beat the Clock
Brilliant Balancers
Chase the Frog

Concentration/Matching Game –
Whole Class

Flower Game

Front to Front

Hoop Game

Jigsaw Game

Knock Down the Tower Game

Ladybird Relaxation

Rainstick Game

Shark Game

Stick Ball Game

Spin the Posture

Two Trees Tag

Yoga Detective What's Missing?

Yoga Relay Game

YEAR 4 (8-9 YEARS)

Beat the Clock

Brilliant Balancers

Chase the Frog

Chips in the Mud

Crown Game

Concentration/Matching Game –
Whole Class

Concentration/Matching Game –
in Small Groups

Dog Relay

Flower Game

Front to Front

Heroes

Hoop Game

Jigsaw Game

Ladybird Relaxation

Make 'Em Laugh

Mixing Game

Posture in the Bag

Queenie, Queenie

Rainstick Game

Shark Game

Sitting on a Chicken

Stick Ball Game

Spin the Posture

The Wrong Posture

Toilet Game

Two Trees Tag

Yoga Detective What's Missing?

Yoga Detective Who's the Leader?

Yoga Relay Game

YEAR 5 (9-10 YEARS)

Beat the Clock

Brilliant Balancers

Butterfly Skittles

Chase the Frog

Chips in the Mud

Crown Game

Concentration/Matching Game –
in Small Groups

Concentration/Matching Game –
Whole Class

Dog Relay

Flower Game

Fleeing Frog

Front to Front

Heroes

Hero in the Corner

Hoop Game

Jigsaw Game

Ladybird Relaxation

Make 'Em Laugh

Mixing Game

One Behind

Poison

Posture in the Bag

Prisoners

Queenie, Queenie

Rainstick Game

Rock Paper Scissors

Sitting on a Chicken

Spin the Posture

Stick Ball Game

The Incredible Weather Game

The Wrong Posture

Three Step Stick

Toilet Game

Two Trees Tag

Yoga Detective What's Missing?

Yoga Detective Who's Talking?

Yoga Detective Who's the Leader?

Yoga Relay Game

Yoglie, Boglie, Moglie

YEAR 6 (10-11 YEARS)

Beat the Clock

Brilliant Balancers

Butterfly Skittles

Chase the Frog

Chips in the Mud

Crown Game

Dog Relay

Flower Game

Fleeing Frog

Front to Front

Heroes

Hero in the Corner

Hoop Game

Jigsaw Game

Ladybird Relaxation

Make 'Em Laugh

Mixing Game

One Behind

Poison

Posture in the Bag

Prisoners

Queenie, Queenie

Rainstick Game

Rock Paper Scissors

Sitting on a Chicken

Stick Ball Game

Spin the Posture

The Incredible Weather Game

The Wrong Posture

Three Step Stick

Toilet Game

Two Trees Tag

Yoga Detective What's Missing?

Yoga Detective Who's Talking?

Yoga Detective Who's the Leader?

Yoga Relay Game

Yoglie, Boglie, Moglie

GAMES BY QUALITIES

Qualities such as assertiveness, awareness, perseverance, taking responsibility and self-control are the pillars of a child's evolving healthy self-esteem. Playing my games will present opportunities to foster those qualities.

ASSERTIVENESS

Flower Game
Hero in the Corner
Jigsaw Game
Rock Paper Scissors
Yoga Detective What's Missing
Yoglie, Boglie, Moglie

AWARENESS

Bean Bag Game (nursery)
Butterfly Skittles
Chase the Frog
Concentration
One Behind
Front to Front
Hero in the Corner
Hoop Game
Matching Game
Poison
Rock Paper Scissors
Shark Game
Spin the Posture

The Incredible Weather Game
Three Step Stick
Umbrella Game (nursery)
What's the Time Mr Wolf?

CALMNESS

Ladybird Relaxation
Matching Game (nursery)
Rainstick Game
Shark Game
Sneaky Trees
What's the Time Mr Wolf?

CREATIVITY

Brilliant Balancers
Concentration
Don't Be Sad
Make 'Em Laugh
Mixing Game
Poison
Sneaky Trees

PERSEVERANCE

Brilliant Balancers
Butterfly Skittles
Dog Relay
Fleeing Frog
Flower Game

Front to Front

Hero in the Corner

Heroes

Hoop Game

Make 'Em Laugh

Matching Game

Mixing Game

One Behind

Queenie, Queenie

Rock Paper Scissors

The Incredible Weather Game

REACTING QUICKLY

Bean Bag Game (nursery)

Beat the Clock

Brilliant Balancers

Butterfly Skittles

Chase the Frog

Chips in the Mud

Don't Be Sad

Fleeing Frog

Hero in the Corner

Heroes

Hoop Game

Make 'Em Laugh

Matching Game (nursery)

Poison

Prisoners

Shark Game

Sneaky Trees

Spin the Posture

The Incredible Weather Game

The Wrong Posture

Three Step Stick

Toilet Game

What's the Time Mr Wolf?

Yoga Detective Who's Leading?

Yoga Relay Game

Yoglie, Boglie, Moglie

SELF-CONTROL

Bean Bag Game (nursery)

Brilliant Balancers

Butterfly Skittles

Concentration

Dog Relay

Fleeing Frog

Flower Game

Front to Front

Hero in the Corner

Heroes

Hoop Game

Jigsaw Game

Ladybird Relaxation

Make 'Em Laugh

Matching Game (nursery)

Mixing Game

Poison

Prisoners

Queenie, Queenie

Rainstick Game

Rock Paper Scissors

Shark Game

Sneaky Trees

Spin the Posture

Stick Ball Game

The Incredible Weather Game

Three Step Stick

Toilet Game

Two Tree Tag

Umbrella Game (nursery)

What's the Time Mr Wolf?

Yoglie, Boglie, Moglie

TAKING RESPONSIBILITY

Chase the Frog
Don't Be Sad
One Behind
Poison
Yoga Detective What's Missing?
Yoga Detective Who's Leading?
Yoga Detective Who's Talking?

GAMES BY SKILLS

My approach has always been that children's yoga, in the form of yoga games, is a vehicle with which children can learn not only important social skills, but also those skills that can increase self-discipline, awareness and control of their bodies. I cannot think of a more fun way to gain such skills other than with games.

BALANCING SKILLS

Brilliant Balancers
Flower Game
Front to Front
Hero in the Corner
Hoop Game
Jigsaw Game
Matching Game (nursery)
Mixing Game
Poison
Prisoners
Rock Paper Scissors
Shark Game
Sneaky Trees
Spin the Posture
Two Tree Tag
Umbrella Game (nursery)
What's the Time Mr Wolf?

CONCENTRATION AND FOCUS

Bean Bag Game (nursery)
Brilliant Balancers
Chase the Frog
Concentration
Crown Game
Flower Game
Front to Front
Hero in the Corner
Hoop Game
Jigsaw Game
Ladybird Relaxation
Matching Game
Matching Game (nursery)
Mixing Game
One Behind
Poison
Prisoners
Queenie, Queenie
Rainstick Game
Rock Paper Scissors
Shark Game
Sneaky Trees
Spin the Posture
Stick Ball Game
The Incredible Weather Game
The Wrong Posture
Three Step Stick
Toilet Game
Two Tree Tag

Umbrella Game (nursery)
What's the Time Mr Wolf?
Yoga Relay Game

DECISION-MAKING

Bean Bag Game (nursery)
Brilliant Balancers
Butterfly Skittles
Chips in the Mud
Concentration
Crown Game
Dog Relay
Don't Be Sad
Fleeing Frog
Flower Game
Front to Front
Hero in the Corner
Heroes
Hoop Game
Matching Game
Mixing Game
Posture in the Bag
Prisoners
Queenie, Queenie
Rainstick Game
Rock Paper Scissors
Shark Game
Stick Ball Game
Spin the Posture
The Incredible Weather Game
Three Step Stick
Umbrella Game (nursery)
Yoga Detective What's Missing?
Yoga Detective Who's Leading?
Yoga Detective Who's Talking?

LISTENING

Brilliant Balancers
Chase the Frog
Flower Game
Ladybird Relaxation
Make 'Em Laugh
Matching Game (nursery)
Mixing Game
One Behind
Poison
Rainstick Game
Rock Paper Scissors
Shark Game
Sneaky Trees
What's the Time Mr Wolf?
Yoga Detective Who's Talking?

OBSERVATIONAL SKILLS

Bean Bag Game (nursery)
Beat the Clock
Brilliant Balancers
Butterfly Skittles
Chase the Frog
Chips in the Mud
Concentration
Crown Game
Fleeing Frog
Flower Game
Front to Front
Hero in the Corner
Heroes
Hoop Game
Jigsaw Game
Ladybird Relaxation
Matching Game

Matching Game (nursery)
One Behind
Poison
Posture in the Bag
Prisoners
Queenie, Queenie
Rainstick Game
Rock Paper Scissors
Shark Game
Sneaky Trees
Spin the Posture
Stick Ball Game
The Incredible Weather Game
Three Step Stick
Toilet Game
Umbrella Game (nursery)
What's the Time Mr Wolf?
Yoga Detective What's Missing?
Yoga Detective Who's Leading?
Yoga Detective Who's Talking?
Yoga Relay Game
Yoglie, Boglie, Moglie

RELAXATION

Bean Bag Game (nursery)
Ladybird Relaxation
Matching Game (nursery)
Sleeping Bird

SEQUENCING

Chase the Frog
One Behind
1. Sun Game
2. Sun Sequence
3. Sun Game in Wheelchairs
4. Sitting Sun Sequence

The Incredible Weather Game
Yoga Detective What's Missing?
Yoga Detective Who's Leading?
Yoga Detective Who's Talking?

SITTING QUIETLY

Bean Bag Game (nursery)
Good Sitting
Knock Down the Tower
Matching Game (nursery)
Rainstick Game
Sitting on a Chicken
Umbrella Game (nursery)

TACTICAL SKILLS

Banana Game
Beat the Clock
Brilliant Balancers
Butterfly Skittles
Chips in the Mud
Concentration
Dog Relay
Fleeing Frog
Flower Game
Front to Front
Hero in the Corner
Heroes
Hoop Game
Make 'Em Laugh
Matching Game
One Behind
Prisoners
Rock Paper Scissors
Shark Game
Stick Ball Game
The Incredible Weather Game

Three Step Stick
Toilet Game
Two Tree Tag
Yoga Detective Who's Leading?
Yoga Detective Who's Talking?
Yoga Relay Game
Yoglie, Boglie, Moglie

TEAMWORK SKILLS

Brilliant Balancers
Butterfly Skittles
Chips in the Mud
Dog Relay
Don't Be Sad
Flower Game
Front to Front
Hero in the Corner
Heroes
Jigsaw Game
Mixing Game
Prisoners
Rock Paper Scissors
Stick Ball Game
Toilet Game
Two Tree Tag
Yoga Relay Game

THINKING

Banana Game
Bean Bag Game (nursery)
Brilliant Balancers
Butterfly Skittles
Chase the Frog
Chips in the Mud
Concentration
Crown Game

Fleeing Frog
Front to Front
Hero in the Corner
Heroes
Hoop Game
Jigsaw Game
Matching Game
Matching Game (nursery)
Mixing Game
One Behind
Poison
Prisoners
Queenie, Queenie
Rainstick Game
Rock Paper Scissors
Shark Game
Sneaky Trees
The Incredible Weather Game
Three Step Stick
Toilet Game
Umbrella Game (nursery)
What's the Time Mr Wolf?
Yoga Detective What's Missing?
Yoga Detective Who's Leading?

USING MATHS

Beat the Clock
Hero in the Corner
Hoop Game

Michael Chissick has been teaching yoga to children in primary mainstream and special needs schools as part of the curriculum for two decades. He is a leading specialist in teaching yoga to children with Autism Spectrum Disorders and continues to train and mentor students who want to teach yoga to children. Michael is the author of *Frog's Breathtaking Speech*, *Ladybird's Remarkable Relaxation*, and *Seahorse's Magical Sun Sequences*, all published by Singing Dragon. Find out more at www.yogaatschool.org.uk.